Rosemary J.N Leicester in 194 slimming club Managing Dir Slimming Clubs.

Also in Arrow by Rosemary Conley

Eat and Stay Slim

EAT YOURSELF SLIM

Rosemary Conley

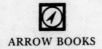

ARROW BOOKS

Arrow Books Limited
17-21 Conway Street, London W1P 6JD

An imprint of the Hutchinson Publishing Group

London Melbourne Sydney Auckland
Johannesburg and agencies throughout
the world

First published in Great Britain by
Hamlyn Paperbacks 1983
Reprinted 1983 (twice)
Arrow edition 1985
Reprinted 1985 (twice)

Printed and bound in Great Britain by
Anchor Brendon Limited, Tiptree, Essex

ISBN 0 09 940620 9

Contents

Foreword

There were all sorts of business reasons why opening slimming clubs for *Successful Slimming* magazine was a good idea. But I knew that the only way we would get them off the ground was with 'the right person' to run them. Everyone I asked said the *only* person would be Rosemary Conley.

I could see what they meant as soon as I met her. First of all, she presented what even our sternest accountants called a 'damn fine' financial plan for the operation (she'd had no experience of this kind of planning) and in spite of considerable scepticism from our friendly but cautious company about the whole idea, Rosemary won them over with her common-sense, unaffected and totally uncomplicated approach to business. (You should have seen this blonde in her business suit and with her huge briefcase handle the pinstripe brigade!)

But they could see – as I could – that she believed *totally* in what she was doing with her own clubs in Leicester. She knew all her staff, she really *loved* her members and revelled in the challenge their weight problems presented. But more than that, she saw them as they were – women battling against the kind of problems only women seem to face: the need to look good, be slim and full of energy and charm whilst juggling kids, husbands, jobs . . . you know the scene.

She arrived at her dieting programme by *personal* trial and error. She put dancing, movement and grooming sessions into her classes because she knew *personally* how boring plain old dieting could be. Even this book came about because she wanted to pass on her own thoughts, ideas and feelings about overweight and dieting – *personally*. As a matter of fact, I first saw the book when it was a much smaller and distinctly less glamorous leaflet she ran off by hand for her own classes.

The really marvellous thing about Rosemary and her crusade for sensible, workable dieting and self-improvement is that success hasn't changed her. She's as excited about the success of the clubs as I am. And we both know they wouldn't be successful if what they do didn't work.

There are, of course, umpteen slimming, diet and exercise books. But not all of them seem to be for people who live in the real world. *Eat Yourself Slim*, on the other hand, relies on what the average British larder contains and makes everyday food into a workable reducing diet. No thinly sliced paw-paws or passion fruits here! The no-nonsense Conley plan drops in the odd packet of Polos, chips and a fresh dollop of cream instead!

If you've been through the slimming mill from starvation to six meals a day, from nothing but eggs and grapefruit to nothing but alcohol or fibre, this book could be your salvation. If I know Rosemary, she'll want to hear from you whatever happens – but I'll bet you'll have only good news to give her from now on!

Jane Reed

Introduction

I believe that most people trying to lose weight eat far too *little* while on their slimming diets – and that they would lose at least as much weight (if not more!) if they ate a *greater* number of calories than most diets allow. Furthermore, by slimming on a higher calorie intake, you'll be much less likely to regain what you have lost once you return to normal eating. Why on earth starve yourself to lose weight, only to put it back on very quickly afterwards? You then feel a total failure, and that's terribly damaging psychologically. We all know that slimming the first time around is relatively easy, whereas subsequent attempts prove more and more difficult.

Having been overweight myself and having tried every type of diet I could get my teeth into, yet still failed to lose weight, I eventually joined a slimming club. I lost my excess weight in a few months but, unfortunately, as soon as I reached my goal weight, I rushed off to eat (in vast quantities!) all the foods which had been banned by the club, with the inevitable result that I regained all the weight I had lost – plus an extra stone (6 kilos)!

I set about diagnosing the situation. I felt strongly that the group therapy method of slimming was a great help, for it was this that had enabled me to find enough willpower to slim when all previous attempts had failed. What, then, was the problem? First, it was too strict, included foods which were expensive and did not fit in with my way of life or my family's. Second, no treats were allowed so quite often I felt hungry and, having once cheated, I couldn't stop myself from continuing to gorge.

So I decided to work out my own plan of action – allowing myself a more generous calorie allowance but working on the principle that, even if it took a little longer, perhaps I wouldn't replace the lost weight after achieving my goal. I joined another slimming club to get the benefit of the group therapy, but I followed *my* diet. To my surprise, I lost weight just as quickly as before and, best of all, I actually *enjoyed* my diet.

Encouraged by this, and becoming more and more fascinated by the subject of slimming as a whole, I studied many aspects of dieting and nutrition and decided to form my own club. This way I could put into practice my theories about slimming and combine them with talks and demonstrations on all aspects of good grooming, which I had learned during a modelling course. I felt it was very important for a slimmer to be able to make the most of her appearance as she lost weight because it was a tremendous help in regaining any confidence lost while being overweight.

I tried out my theories on six of my neighbours – and the medically-approved diets worked splendidly! Then I opened a club, to which members of the public were invited, and 29 eager slimmers joined. In less than seven years, the membership of my slimming club had grown to over 15,000 – and that was just in Leicestershire.

In October 1980 I was invited to London by Jane Reed, who was at the time the publisher of *Successful Slimming* magazine. I was asked if I thought similar clubs to mine could be organised throughout the country in association with *Successful Slimming* magazine – a publication which Jane Reed had originally created. I knew that my theories worked – after all, I had 15,000 successful slimmers to prove it. I had trained a team of lecturers who were excellent at their job, so I could see no reason why this should not be extended. It was all very exciting and an enormous challenge.

We now have over fifty fully-trained Area Managers plus hundreds of lecturers – including dieticians, corsetières, beauticians, graduates, nurses, and hairdressers (all of whom have experienced a previous weight problem) – who take between them hundreds of SSAGG classes every week all over the United Kingdom. These classes include slimming, good grooming and exercises practised to popular music. I also take my own classes. We also run a postal course with members all over Great Britain.

It is our philosophy to encourage the new slimmer to consume the maximum calories which will still enable her to lose weight, usually between 1,400 and 1,600 calories per day. After a week, they can't believe they have actually lost weight! Comments such as 'I've eaten more on this diet than I did before' are commonplace. And not only do they lose weight, but they lose *lots* of weight – 10 pounds (4.5 kilos), is not unusual!

One day recently a desperately unhappy lady rang me, saying that she was beside herself with worry about her weight, but that while she was really keen to attend one of our classes, she dreaded being the fattest there. She weighed over 20 stones (127 kilos) and felt embarrassed to go out at all, let alone to a meeting where she felt she would be the star attraction! I told her that we loved having someone with plenty of weight to lose because it offered us a challenge – and that many people felt just as desperate with only 2 stones (12.5 kilos) to lose. She finally agreed to go along to a nearby class that evening. I asked her if she would begin her diet on 1,700 calories a day, so that we would have plenty of room for reducing her calories later on if necessary. Because I was so interested in her particular weight problem she also agreed to write down everything she ate, recording the calorie content alongside.

By the following Tuesday, Mary had already lost 1st 2lb (7.25 kilos). She was over the moon – as was everyone else in her class, knowing very well how much courage she had shown in joining. Pat, the marvellous lecturer in charge of Mary's class, kept me informed of her progress. Unfortunately, like many slimmers, Mary had been impatient and, after a couple of weeks, admitted to eating only 1,300 calories a day. I was sorry because I felt she would probably have lost almost as much weight during that first week on the higher intake.

However, after five weeks we did manage to persuade

Mary to try eating 1,500 calories and to her amazement – though not to ours – she lost 4 pounds (1.75 kilos) compared with only half that during the previous week. She then decided to trust us and increased her intake to 1,650 calories. In 14 weeks her weight loss totalled 4 st 9 lb (29.5 kilos). She is continuing on around 1,500 calories now and loses 3-4 pounds (1.5-1.75 kilos) weekly. I have Mary's diet sheets showing every single mouthful she has eaten during the last few months and at the time of writing this book, Mary has lost 5 st (32 kilos) in 17 weeks. She looks and feels years younger – and is really beginning to live again.

I hope Mary's experiences will offer encouragement to the readers of this book, which is based on my own experience of slimming successfully – I now weigh 8 stone (51 kilos) – and of helping many thousands of other previously-failed slimmers to reach their goal . . . and remain slim!

I do hope that my diets and theories – plus quite a few hints and recipes – will help you achieve *your* ideal weight.

Good Luck!

Rosemary J.N. Conley

1

How Much Can I Eat And Still Lose Weight?

I think it would be sensible to clarify the meaning of two words which are used constantly in connection with slimming – 'calorie' and 'metabolism'.

Calories

Most people know that a calorie is a unit of heat (and therefore energy). The amount of heat produced by a piece of coal is measured in calories and, similarly, our bodies burn food which produces heat or energy. Generally speaking, if we consume more calories than we burn, we store the excess in the form of fat and we gain weight. If our calorie intake equals our energy output our weight remains constant – but if we wish to reduce weight, we must eat fewer calories than we burn. That's when our bodies draw on reserve stores of fat. However, it is essential to eat sufficient of the right sort of food while dieting to remain in good health.

Metabolic rate

Metabolism is the word used to describe the change of food into the chemical constituents the body needs to exist and grow. Metabolic rate is the rate at which one's body burns fuel or, to compare a human body with a motor car, one's rate of miles per gallon! Some people are fortunate enough to be able to eat anything and have their weight remain constant, while others seem to gain weight after eating just one good meal in a restaurant.

Let's compare the person who can eat anything, yet maintains a constant weight, with a Rolls Royce motor car. This magnificent vehicle consumes a considerable amount of petrol on a given journey compared with, say, a Mini, which will go the same distance on remarkably less fuel. Those of us who gain weight easily are, regrettably, like the Mini. When extra supplies of fuel are delivered, extra fuel tanks have to be built in order to store the fuel. These stores are, in human terms, fat cells.

We cannot change the way we are made – so we must accept our 'styling' and, if we are to stop our fat stores increasing, we must stop the deliveries of fuel which are surplus to our requirements. In the short term, it is also necessary to cut back on our intake in order to use up some of the accumulated stores.

The basal metabolic rate of an average female is approximately 1,400 calories per day – this is the number of calories she burns up in keeping her body mechanism ticking over. As soon as she starts any physical activity, she uses more fuel and therefore burns up more calories.

A mother with three young children under school age, a husband and a home to look after, a dog to exercise regularly and no car in which to go shopping, would be classed as very active. She would probably burn in the region of 2,500 calories per day.

A mother with two school-age children, a part-time clerical job at which she sits down most of the time and a husband who dines out at lunchtime, might be classed as moderately active. She would probably burn around 2,000–2,200 calories per day.

But many women do not fall into either category and must be classed as inactive. This does not necessarily mean that they are ladies of leisure – far from it. Such a person could be a hard-working woman in a high-powered job – but most of her exertion would be in *mental* activity. Unfortunately, brain work doesn't burn up very many calories! Our career woman probably has her own car and, because of her life style, probably doesn't have time to go shopping every day. She therefore organises herself into a weekly – or even a monthly – shopping routine. Her freezer is well stocked, her washing may be sent to the laundry and the dishwasher cleans the dishes. She may also have cleaning help in the home. Because of the very demanding nature of her work, our career woman frequently comes home in the evenings feeling totally exhausted. She may watch television or read a book because she needs to relax in this way to relieve the mental stress of the office day. It is not surprising that she has little energy left for physical exercise.

A more usual 'sedentary' existence is that of the woman whose children have grown up and left home, and who has only her husband and home to care for. The rush has gone out of her life and she can take her time. As she gets older she will move about less quickly so that her calorie/energy output is inevitably lower. It is estimated that a woman in a sedentary situation burns approximately 1,800–2,000 calories per day.

It may surprise you to learn that there is a very narrow margin between each of these categories. But it must be understood that the bulk of energy/calorie output is expended in the maintenance and running of our bodies, not in the physical or mental activity they are asked to perform. To further illustrate this point, to burn up a pound (0.5 kilo) of fat by physical exercise alone you would need to walk approximately 50 miles (80 kilometres)!

It is now accepted that exercise and activity alone are not effective ways of reducing weight – but exercise is extremely good for almost everyone and will certainly help to tone your body while you are reducing your weight. (See Exercise chapter, page 68). It will also promote better health.

Working out your daily calorie allowance

Hopefully you will now have some idea of your calorie/energy output, so we must arrive at a level of calorie intake which will effect a significant weight loss but allow you as much food as possible to avoid getting hungry. If you enjoy your diet and never feel hungry, your chances of keeping to it are considerably greater!

When you embark on a reducing diet, the area of your body is at its greatest. As it reduces in size, it obviously requires less fuel to maintain it. So after shedding a stone (6 kilos) or so, your body may not reduce its weight on the

15

calorie allowance with which you started your slimming campaign. Should you wish to reduce your weight further, a reduction in your daily calorie intake of approximately 200 would soon effect acceptable weight losses again. Continue on this lower calorie intake until your body reaches another plateau after losing another 1½-2 stones (8.5-12.5 kilos), then again reduce your daily allowance.

In my experience I have found that slimmers reach a plateau whether they start on 1,000 calories a day or 1,600 calories a day. The poor 1,000-a-day slimmer is going to feel ravenous on the 700 calories to which she may find she has to reduce, in order to shift those last few pounds (or kilos). On the other hand, with my method of maximum calories, no one need ever fall below a daily intake of 1,000 calories. In fact, I would definitely advise that they should not!

The following table illustrates the ideal calorie intake according to your activity rating – and keep to the maximum calorie allowance for as long as possible. Only reduce your calorie intake if no weight loss has occurred for at least two weeks. Always take the next lower rating; *never* try to take short cuts to an even lower calorie allowance.

	Estimated energy/ calorie output	Initial calorie allowance	Reducing calorie allowances		
			1st	2nd	Final
Women					
Very active	2,500	1,700	1,500	1,300	1,150
Active	2,200	1,600	1,400	1,250	1,100
Moderately active	2,000	1,500	1,300	1,150	1,050
Sedentary	1,800-2,000	1,400	1,200	1,100	1,000
Men					
Very active	3,500-4,000	2,500	2,200	2,000	1,800
Active	3,000-3,350	2,100	1,950	1,750	1,650
Moderately active	2,700	1,900	1,800	1,650	1,550
Sedentary	2,500	1,800	1,700	1,600	1,500

Anyone who is grossly overweight should increase the above allowances as follows:

Stones (kilos) overweight	Extra daily calorie allowance
3 (19)	50
4 (25.5)	100
5 (32)	150
6 (38)	200
7 (44.5)	250
8 (51)	300
9 (57)	350
10 (63.5)	400

Slimming on the maximum number of calories

Remember, it is advisable to consult your doctor before embarking on a reducing diet – particularly if you have in excess of a stone (6 kilos) to lose. But argue if he says you should stick to 1,000 calories per day. I promise you that 99 people out of every 100 who are overweight will lose weight more effectively on a considerably higher intake and are far less likely to regain their lost weight.

To illustrate my point, let me tell you some success stories!

Recently one of my lecturers informed me of the success of Sonia, who had joined one of our classes a month previously, weighing in at 15 stones (95.5 kilos). She is a tall girl, leading a moderately active life and from the day she joined our class she kept rigidly to our 1,450-calorie diet. In four weeks she had shed 1½ stones (8.5 kilos)!

Another member, Pam, lost 5 stones (32 kilos) in six months on the same diet in 1976. She reduced from a dress size 24 to dress size 12 and has maintained her goal weight ever since.

Jean weighed 13 st 3 lb (84 kilos) when she joined one of my classes in May, having lost 3 st 4 lb (21 kilos) previously. I suggested a 1,400-calorie diet, despite the fact that she had been on a lower calorie intake. Her weight continued to reduce even on this higher allowance and by August Jean had lost another stone (6 kilos)!

In September I reduced Jean's allowance to 1,200 and by October she was down to 10 st 12 lbs (69 kilos). Again we reduced the calorie allowance, this time to 1,000 calories, and by November Jean weighed 10 st 7 lb (67 kilos), her goal weight. Six months later Jean was able to eat whatever she liked without gaining, providing she didn't grossly *overeat*.

A few weeks after reaching her goal, I thought it would be interesting to see how many calories Jean was consuming as she was now eating normally. I asked her to write down every single thing that she ate during the next seven days, to weigh everything and to calculate the calorie values. The daily average amounted to 1,800 and that week she lost half a pound (225 grams)!

This emphasises the other important reason for slimming on the maximum number of calories - that after reducing your weight to the desired level you will be able to eat normally again without regaining the weight you've lost!

When I say that a few weeks or months after achieving your goal weight you will be able to eat normally, I mean that you may rely on your natural appetite to direct you towards a sensible level of intake. I do not mean that you will be able to eat a whole packet of chocolate biscuits followed by fish and chips! That is gluttony, not sensible eating! You have to learn that you can't have your cake and eat it twice!

For some reason our bodies adjust after a period of time to a certain level of calorie intake, whether it be 1,400, 1,000 or even 700 calories. Only by gradually increasing the fuel intake by 100-200 at a time over a period of a few weeks will our bodies adjust to accept the fuel without storing it as unwanted fat. I also believe that the maximum increase possible, over a period of months, without your weight increasing, is 600 calories. Therefore, given time and patience, someone dieting on 1,400 calories will ultimately maintain a constant weight on 2,000 calories, whereas someone who reduced to a consumption of 700 calories would never hope to maintain their weight on more than 1,300 calories - which is nowhere near 'normal' eating!

By following the diets suggested in this book, you will find that your appetite becomes educated towards sensible eating.

The following is a typical case history:
Commencing weight: 15 stones (95.5 kilos)
Age of subject: 43 years
Desired goal weight: 10 stones (63.5 kilos)
Activity group: Moderately active
Initial calorie allowance: 1,650

	Weight	Calorie intake
After 1 month	14 stones (89 kilos)	1,650
2 months	13st 6lb (85.5 kilos)	1,650
3 months	13st 2lb (83.5 kilos)	1,650
Calorie allowance reduced to: 1,450		
4 months	12st 7lb (79.5 kilos)	1,450
5 months	12st 1lb (77 kilos)	1,450
Calorie allowance reduced to: 1,250		
6 months	11st 4lb (72 kilos)	1,250
7 months	10st 9lb (67.5 kilos)	1,250
Calorie allowance reduced to: 1,100		
8 months	10 stones (63.5 kilos) goal weight	
Calorie allowance increased to: 1,300		
9 months	9st 12lb (62.5 kilos)	1,300
Calorie allowance increased to: 1,500		
10 months	9st 12lb (62.5 kilos)	1,500
Calorie allowance increased to: 1,700		
11 months	9st 12lb (62.5 kilos)	1,700
Calorie allowance increased to: 1,800		
12 months	9st 12lb (62.5 kilos) normal eating	

Our subject found that if she over-ate one day she automatically cut down the next day. The 'normal eating' allowance for her varied from 1,700 to 2,000 calories per day.

When you have achieved your weight goal and are managing to keep your weight reasonably stable by eating sensibly, you will be able to enjoy a more relaxed attitude towards your food and fluid intake. This will make life much more enjoyable and you will gain more and more confidence in your ability to control your eating habits. The panic experienced by dieters who go 'off the rails' soon disappears.

Your ideal weight

You will not find an 'ideal weight' chart in this book as I do not believe in them. *You* know whether or not you are overweight just by looking at yourself in the mirror with no clothes on!

Recommended weights can vary so much according to bone structure, etc., that few people are able to calculate accurately their own 'ideal' weight. They often add a little to their height to take them into the next weight bracket and then feel delighted to read that their weight is said to be 'ideal'! But the midriff bulge is still there and so are the heavy, bulging thighs etc.

Your ideal weight is the weight at which you look your most attractive, though this may be half a stone (3 kilos) heavier or lighter than is recommended by the charts.

Speed of weight loss

Before embarking on any form of reducing diet, you must realise that to lose weight your body must burn up some of its reserves which are stored in the form of fat. There is obviously a limit to how fast this can be done and you must accept the fact that a certain amount of patience is needed for you to reach your desired weight.

Crash diets are a complete waste of time and I do not propose to waste space discussing them. However, an occasional one-day fast or a very low-calorie day following an over-eating spell can prove to be invaluable. This aspect will be dealt with under Binge Eating (see page 63).

I am always being asked how quickly people can lose weight on my diets. I can only say that different people react in different ways on different diets – but if the suggested diets are adhered to totally, weight loss can be considerable.

Occasionally, quite early on in your dieting campaign, you may find that your weight remains constant even though you have been particularly strict with yourself. This is a peculiarity of the human body and is completely beyond our control. If you have not adhered to your present calorie allowance for very long, please do not reduce it further as it may not be the calorie intake that has produced the plateau, but possibly fluid level variation. Continue with your diet regardless, taking particular care to count every mouthful. Soon your body will regulate itself once more and you will again see a reduction in your weight.

Many women find that a significant weight gain occurs just prior to a menstrual period – an increase of as much as 6 pounds (2.75 kilos) is not unusual. However, some women experience no such increase at their period but at some other time during their menstrual cycle, at a regular time each month. Also many women find dieting difficult prior to menstruation as they often feel very low or depressed. If you suffer in this way, it would be sensible to anticipate a possible lack of willpower at this time and so allow a more generous diet, trying also to busy yourself with some hobby that you enjoy.

2

Practical Nutrition

Diets are often designed by nutritional specialists who formulate eating plans based on text book dietetics with little thought to practical eating. Such a diet might include steamed smoked haddock and watercress for breakfast; cottage cheese, salad, crispbread plus an apple for lunch, and braised kidneys, tomatoes, peas and a small potato plus an orange for the evening meal. There would most likely be a daily allowance of 300ml/½ pint milk and 15g/½ oz butter.

While I admit that this is a highly nutritious diet, I would consider the following to be far more attractive to the average female dieter:

Breakfast	small glass unsweetened orange juice or
	½ fresh grapefruit
	2 grilled tomatoes with 25g/1oz grilled lean bacon
	25g/1oz toast, butter from daily allowance,
	1 teaspoon marmalade
Lunch	75g/3oz lean red meat or 100g/4oz poultry
	100g/4oz sliced beans, 100g/4oz carrots,
	50g/2oz new potatoes, thin gravy
	fresh fruit salad and 25ml/1fl oz single cream
Dinner	50g/2oz toast
	25g/1oz hard cheese
	1 poached egg
	1 tomato
	100g/4oz stewed fruit (no sugar)
Daily allowance	300ml/½ pint milk
	15g/½ oz butter
	treat of your choice, amounting to no more than
	100 calories

Total calories for the day: 1,400

With this specimen menu, it might be preferable to save certain items until later in the day, particularly if you are an 'evening nibbler'. For example, you could save the toast and marmalade from breakfast and the fresh fruit salad and cream from lunch. It may also suit you to split the evening meal into two smaller meals,

6 pm   Poached egg on toast, fruit
9 pm   Cheese and tomato sandwich

If you are out at work all day, you may need to take a packed lunch. By re-organising the day's ingredients you could produce a very substantial packed lunch, leaving your main meal for the evening when you return home. All that is necessary is for you to save your bread allowance from breakfast and combine it with the 50g/2oz bread allowed for the evening meal, then make cheese and tomato and egg and tomato sandwiches. You could take a fresh apple or pear to complete your packed lunch. Your treat could, of course, be taken at any time.

You must make a diet fit in to *your* way of living. However, I cannot stress too much the absolute necessity for your diet to be nutritionally sound. If it is deficient in almost anything, you could soon begin to feel lethargic, tired and irritable.

I do not propose to write at length on the subject of nutrition, as there are excellent books available which deal with it in great detail – but it would be foolhardy to write a book about slimming without explaining the basic requirements for healthy eating.

Nutrients and their sources
Foods contain five types of nutrients:
Proteins which help to build body cells and also supply energy.
Carbohydrates and *Fats* which supply energy; this also includes alcohol.
Minerals which help to build some parts of the body, protect it from deficiency diseases and regulate metabolism.
Vitamins which help to regulate metabolism and protect the body from deficiency diseases.

Proteins

Protein-containing foods are meat, fish, eggs and cheese, but milk, baked beans, pulse vegetables, soya flour, Textured Vegetable Protein, wholemeal bread and nuts are also rich sources of this vital nutrient. Protein-rich food satisfies you for longer than carbohydrate-rich food, therefore avoiding premature hunger-pangs, so it is advisable to consume some protein-rich food with each meal – with an absolute minimum of two average helpings a day.

If you are a vegetarian, it is important that you take time and trouble to ensure that your diet contains sufficient of these foods.

Carbohydrates

These can be separated into two categories – good ones and bad ones! Carbohydrates are necessary to provide energy, and good sources of carbohydrates are bread, potatoes, rice, pasta and flour. They are good because they contain many other nutrients as well as carbohydrates. However, we can well do without the bad carbohydrates (often rich in sugar) like jam, treacle, sweets, chocolates, sweetened squashes, fizzy drinks etc. These foods are all sources of 'empty' calories and are also bad for your teeth. When dieting, it is wise to take the foods listed under 'good' in moderation and those listed under 'bad' only very occasionally but preferably not at all!

Fats

Small amounts are essential to good health. As well as being found in butter, margarine, cooking oil, lard, dripping and cream, fat is also found in egg yolk, cheese, fatty meat and fatty fish. Ounce for ounce fat provides the highest number of calories compared with any other food – 226 per oz (25g) – so it is obvious that the dieter must be careful not to over-indulge in this direction.

Minerals

Iron and calcium are minerals essential to healthy living. Iron is needed particularly by women as it is the nutrient required to make haemoglobin of blood and a deficiency would produce anaemia. Women lose blood during menstruation so it is most important that their diet contains an adequate ration of iron. Foods rich in iron are liver and kidney, but red meat, egg yolk, dark green vegetables and cocoa are valuable sources too. Our bodies make more use of the iron in vegetables if we take it with Vitamin C (eg orange or grapefruit or pure lemon juice).

We need calcium for healthy bones and teeth, and it is found in milk, cheese, yoghurt, tinned fish and dark green vegetables. It is also added to white bread and white flour.

Vitamins

There are two types of vitamin: water soluble and fat soluble. Water soluble vitamins must be consumed daily as they cannot be stored in the body, whereas fat soluble vitamins can be stored, so daily consumption is not essential.

Vitamin A is a fat soluble vitamin which helps to give a healthy skin and also helps our eyesight. It is found in margarine, liver, cod liver oil, cheese, butter, eggs, kidneys, carrots, spinach, watercress and tomato.

Vitamin D is also a fat soluble vitamin and it works with calcium in the formation of healthy bones and teeth. Vitamin D is found in margarine, eggs, milk (particularly evaporated), fatty fish and cod liver oil. The sun's rays fall on to the skin and convert a substance in our bodies into Vitamin D; we should therefore expose ourselves as often as possible to the sunshine.

B Vitamins are water soluble. The B complex is a group of 13 chemically unrelated substances. Basically Vitamin B is necessary to the nervous system and should never be neglected. It is found in wheat flour, Marmite, liver, cheese, eggs, milk, oatmeal, green peas and bacon. Wholemeal bread is a rich source of Vitamin B and should be chosen in preference to white bread, though these days white bread does have added vitamins.

Vitamin C is also water soluble. It helps us to resist infection and is found in fresh and frozen fruit and vegetables, especially citrus fruits, fruit juices, tomatoes and green vegetables. However, Vitamin C is easily destroyed by over-cooking, keeping the food warm or by adding bicarbonate of soda during cooking. Storing fresh vegetables for several days also causes loss of vitamin content. It is therefore a good idea to eat plenty of raw vegetables whenever possible and to shop regularly to ensure fresh supplies.

Fibre in the diet

A common complaint of the dieter is constipation. This is caused by the reduction of fibre in the diet brought about by avoiding such foods as bread and potatoes. We need fibre to enable our bowels to work properly and, as the present trend is to use convenience foods made from white flour, constipation is becoming an increasing problem.

As fibre also helps you to feel full yet contains few calories, it is important to realise where fibre-rich foods may be found. Wholemeal bread is an excellent source of fibre and it will satisfy you far more than white bread. Bran breakfast cereals and natural bran are all rich in fibre. For the slimmer, particularly, natural bran from a health store or your local chemist is the best solution to constipation. Introduce pure bran into your diet gradually by taking 1 teaspoon on the first day, 2 teaspoons on the second day and so on until you find the correct level of intake to effect a satisfactory bowel movement. It is best taken with a little milk, in fruit juice, tomato juice, natural yoghurt or sprinkled on to cereals, soups, stews or gravy. Fibre is also to be found in vegetables and fruit. Potatoes in jackets and apples and pears with the peel kept on are ideal. It is essential to take plenty of fluids to help 'move' the fibre.

Making up your own diet

One food which we do not need is sugar as it contains no proteins or vitamins whatsoever, so avoid it whenever possible. When you are dieting, remember to eat all foods in moderation and that variety is essential. Eat at least three meals a day including breakfast or mid-morning snack.

If you wish to make up your own diet, each day must contain:

2-3 average helpings of high-protein foods
At least 2 helpings of fresh or frozen vegetables
At least 2 helpings of fresh fruit
Moderate amounts of wholemeal bread and potatoes
Small amount of fat

26

300ml/½ pint fresh milk (or 600ml/1 pint skimmed milk)
Drink at least 1.15 litres/2 pints of fluid (not alcohol unless
   allowed on diet) every day

3

What Makes A Good Diet?

A good diet is a diet which is successful. For it to be successful:

1   It must be nutritionally sound.
2   It must appeal to you.
3   It must fit in with your life style.
4   There must be a margin of freedom allowing you a treat of your choice.
5   It must contain enough food to prevent you from feeling hungry.
6   It must be flexible so that dining out can be enjoyable.
7   It should contain everyday foods and avoid additional expense.
8   It should be adaptable so that the rest of the family may be fed on similar food.
9   It should contain plenty of variety.
10 It should contain foods that you enjoy eating.

You may feel that this list of requirements would be impossible to find – but I assure you that it *is* possible to find the perfect diet for *you*.

On the pages that follow you will find several very different diets. They have all been exhaustively tested for their effectiveness. They have also all been examined and found to be nutritionally sound in their composition.

Before each diet I offer a brief explanation as to its why's and wherefore's, and I hope you will find this helpful.

Diet No 1   **1,400-Calorie Diet (Women)**
This is the main diet recommended to those who join my

slimming classes and thousands of women have slimmed extremely successfully on it. I have witnessed weight losses of up to a stone (6 kilos) in the first week – though the average is more likely to be 5-7 pounds (2.25-3.25 kilos) – and a weekly loss of 2-4 pounds (1-1.75 kilos) is usually experienced thereafter.

For those who should consume in excess of 1,400 calories because of the amount of weight to be lost or their activity rating, the extra calories may be consumed in any way they wish.

Most women should lose weight if their daily intake is restricted to 1,400 calories. This diet has been designed to fit into your family's way of eating and no one need guess that you are dieting.

You may change meals around within each day but try to keep to one day at a time. In other words, don't use Wednesday's breakfast, Friday's lunch and Tuesday's evening meal to make up one day's eating. Each day has been designed to incorporate the necessary foods for a balanced diet.

On Sunday, Monday and Wednesday 50 calories are left over, and on Tuesday, Thursday, Friday and Saturday 150 calories remain. Below are a few suggestions for using them up:

50 calories (approximately)

1 plain sweet biscuit	1 large apple
1 orange	1 large pear
100g/4oz grapes	50g/2oz banana
25g/1oz ice cream	1 teaspoon marmalade
1 small glass dry sherry	1 small glass gin
1 small glass wine	

150 calories (approximately)

300ml/½ pint beer	2 whiskies or other spirits
300ml/½ pint fresh milk (additional to allowance)	25g/1oz chocolate
	1 150g/5oz carton flavoured yoghurt
2 tablespoons extra thick fresh cream	1 small portion of apple pie
1 doughnut	65g/2½ oz ice cream
25g/1oz bread with 7g/¼ oz butter	1 small piece of cake

If you find yourself really hungry and with very few calories left from your daily allowance, the following are recommended: raw carrot, sticks of celery or clear home-made soup.

Note Weights quoted for meats, etc. are the cooked weights.

600ml/1 pint skimmed milk may be substituted for 300ml/½ pint fresh milk.

25g/1oz low-fat spread may be used in place of 15g/½ oz butter.

Low-calorie salad dressing may be used instead of ordinary salad cream. Double the amount, eg. 1 tablespoon salad cream or 2 tablespoons low-calorie salad dressing.

1 slice bread – 25g/1oz (wholemeal is preferable); 1 potato (size of an egg) – 50g/2oz.

Add chopped raw onion or green peppers to your cottage cheese to make it more tasty.

Don't worry if you miss a meal – you won't starve!

To be consumed daily
300ml/½ pint fresh milk
15g/½ oz butter or margarine
Drinks may be taken mid-morning, mid-afternoon and evening using milk from daily allowance. Slimline and low-calorie drinks may be taken freely.

SUNDAY
Breakfast
½ grapefruit
25g/1oz wholemeal bread
cup of tea or coffee

Lunch
100g/4oz roast meat
100g/4oz green vegetables
1 jacket potato
a little gravy
100g/4oz fresh fruit salad (no sugar)

Dinner

salad with 100g/4oz cottage cheese or 25g/1oz hard cheese or 50g/2oz sliced ham

1 tablespoon salad cream or 2 tablespoons low-calorie salad dressing

1 apple or pear

MONDAY
Breakfast

drink of honey and hot water plus a slice of lemon

1 scrambled egg

25g/1oz wholemeal toast

2 slices tomato

Lunch

250ml/8oz soup (medium thick)

1 egg omelette with large salad of lettuce, cucumber, onion and tomato

low-calorie salad dressing if required

Dinner

100g/4oz lean meat or offal

100g/4oz green vegetable or salad

50g/2oz jacket potato

100g/4oz fresh fruit salad

TUESDAY
Breakfast

½ grapefruit

25g/1oz grilled lean bacon

1 fried egg cooked in very little fat

15g/½ oz wholemeal bread

Lunch

salad of lettuce, cucumber, slice of onion, grated carrot, tomato plus 100g/4oz cottage cheese *or* 25g/1oz hard cheese

1 pear

Dinner

175g/6oz grilled plaice

100g/4oz French or runner beans

50g/2oz chips

1 Slimline jelly (see page 87)

WEDNESDAY

Breakfast

½ grapefruit
1 boiled egg
25g/1oz wholemeal bread

Lunch

25g/1oz wholemeal bread
40g/1½ oz hard cheese, toasted, garnished with 1 tomato
1 apple
1 pear

Dinner

150ml/¼ pint thin soup
1 grilled lean lamb chop
50g/2oz jacket potato
100g/4oz carrots
100g/4oz cabbage or beans
1 orange

THURSDAY

Breakfast

1 small carton natural yoghurt with 1 teaspoon pure honey
   and 1 teaspoon chopped nuts
   OR
1 whole grapefruit and 1 boiled egg

Lunch

50g/2oz wholemeal bread made into a sandwich with 25g/
   1oz hard cheese, 1 tomato, lettuce, cucumber and 1 teaspoon salad cream
1 orange

Dinner

4 fish fingers, grilled
75g/3oz peas
100g/4oz green beans
50g/2oz chips
1 tablespoon tomato ketchup, if liked
50g/2oz grapes
1 apple

FRIDAY
Breakfast
small glass unsweetened fruit juice
25g/1oz grilled lean bacon
15g/½ oz wholemeal bread
2 tomatoes, grilled

Lunch
100g/4oz cottage cheese with lettuce, tomato, cucumber, onion, grated carrot
1 hard-boiled egg
1 tablespoon salad cream or 2 tablespoons low-calorie salad dressing
1 apple or pear

Dinner
100g/4oz chicken
50g/2oz jacket potato
100g/4oz cabbage
100g/4oz green beans
a little gravy
1 orange

SATURDAY
Breakfast
cup of coffee
1 apple and 1 orange or 1 whole grapefruit
25g/1oz grilled lean bacon
2 tomatoes, grilled

Lunch
2 beefburgers
1 tomato
50g/2oz mushrooms
1 fried egg
100g/4oz green vegetable
50g/2oz chips
Slimline jelly (see page 87)

Dinner
1 boiled egg
25g/1oz wholemeal bread
tomato
1 piece fruit

Diet No 2   1,800-Calorie Diet (Men)

For men to lose weight successfully, their diet must be practical. This 1,800-calorie eating programme offers a selection of meals from which any overweight man should be able to select an acceptable menu.

When I formulated this diet, I endeavoured to design a selection of menus which would cover all possible eating situations, eg. the pub lunch, meals in canteens, cafés and restaurants, packed lunches, etc. The daily 'treat' allowance of 250 calories should be adequate to cover the odd drink. Anyone who enjoys a 'night out with the lads' could save his week's treat calories for his one night out:

7 × 250 = 1,750 calories, which means 7-11 pints (4-6 litres) beer (depending on the brand). Surely that's enough for anyone! Certainly your friends won't guess that you are dieting if you don't want them to.

The calorie allowance for each meal is indicated so that should the dieter dine out and one of our meal suggestions is not available, he should be able to calculate the calorie values of the food consumed and make any necessary adjustment at a later stage in the day.

I have found that men respond very favourably to this diet, losing about a stone (6 kilos) a month on average.

Diet rules
You are allowed three meals a day. In addition to these you are allowed 250 calories which may be used as you wish. The meals may be eaten at any time.

The calorie values of the meals are as follows:

Breakfast	250 calories
Lunch	600 calories
Dinner	550 calories
Snack	250 calories

Additionally, you are allowed 300ml/½ pint fresh milk daily, or 600ml/1 pint skimmed milk.

Tea and coffee may be drunk freely, provided that your milk allowance is not exceeded, and that artificial sweeteners are used in place of sugar. Low-calorie squashes, slimline drinks, pure lemon juice and water are also unrestricted.

Breakfasts

1 ½ grapefruit, 1 boiled egg, 25g/1oz wholemeal bread, 15g/½oz low-fat spread, 15g/½oz marmalade.

2 ½ grapefruit, 25g/1oz grilled lean bacon, 1 fried egg, 15g/½oz wholemeal bread.

3 90ml/3 fl oz unsweetened orange juice, 25g/1oz Special K, 7g/¼oz sugar, 150ml/¼ pint milk.

4 90ml/3 fl oz unsweetened orange juice, 2 Weetabix, 7g/¼oz sugar, 150ml/¼ pint milk.

Lunches

1 300ml/½ pint clear soup, 100g/4oz roast lean meat or 175g/6oz chicken, 75g/3oz potatoes (jacket or boiled), 175g/6oz green vegetables, 75g/3oz carrots, 2 tablespoons thin gravy. Piece of fruit.

2 1 fried egg, 100g/4oz chips, 2 large grilled sausages, 50g/2oz peas. Small portion ice cream.

3 2 cheese or salad rolls and 600ml/1 pint any beer.

4 4 thin slices from large wholemeal loaf made into sandwiches with salad filling and spread with low-fat spread and a little low-calorie salad dressing *plus* 1 hard-boiled egg or 25g/1oz hard cheese. Piece of fruit or 150g/5oz carton natural yoghurt.

Dinners

1 175ml/6 fl oz thick soup. Large salad comprising lettuce, tomatoes, cucumber, celery, spring onions, grated carrot, beetroot, 1 hard-boiled egg *plus* 75g/3oz cold lean meat or 100g/4oz chicken or 30g/2oz cheese. 100g/4oz stewed fruit (no sugar).

2 Grilled lean pork chop (50g/2oz cooked weight), 75g/3oz jacket potato, 175g/6oz green vegetables, 75g/3oz carrots, little thin gravy. 1 baked apple sweetened with artificial sweetener and 1 tablespoon single cream.

3   225g/8oz steamed or grilled haddock (175g/6oz with breadcrumbs or batter), 75g/3oz chips, 100g/4oz sliced green beans. 50g/2oz fruit pie.
4   50g/2oz liver, 50g/2oz lean bacon, 1 large sausage (all grilled), 100g/4oz green vegetables, 25g/1oz potato. 50g/2oz ice cream.

Diet No 3   1,200-Calorie Diet (Women)

This diet should be attempted only after you have been on a higher calorie diet, ie. 1,400+ calories per day, and have reached a plateau.

DO NOT TAKE SHORT CUTS BY *STARTING* YOUR SLIMMING CAMPAIGN ON THIS DIET!

After one week of following this diet, change to the next 1,200-calorie diet. You will now have been dieting for some time and variety is of the utmost importance.

300ml/½ pint fresh milk to be consumed daily (drinks may be taken when desired using milk from allowance).

MONDAY

Breakfast

15g/½ oz Special K or 1 Weetabix plus milk from allowance
1 teaspoon sugar

Lunch

100g/4oz roast chicken
100g/4oz cabbage
75g/3oz carrots
2 small pieces of roast potato
little gravy
Lemon meringue pie (see page 88)

Dinner

lettuce, cucumber, ½ hard-boiled egg, grated raw carrot
100g/4oz cottage cheese with 1 tomato, slice onion, celery
15g/½ oz wholemeal bread
7g/¼ oz butter or 15g/½ oz low-fat spread
1 teaspoon salad cream

TUESDAY
Breakfast
25g/1oz lean grilled bacon
2 tomatoes, grilled
15g/½ oz wholemeal bread

Lunch
½ grapefruit
salad with 25g/1oz grated cheese
1 teaspoon salad cream
100g/4oz grapes or 1 orange

Dinner
300ml/½ pint clear soup
Grilled lean pork chop weighing 100g/4oz on bone (no fat)
50g/2oz apple sauce (no sugar)
100g/4oz green beans
3oz peas
50g/2oz jacket potato
7g/¼ oz butter or 15g/½ oz low-fat spread
Lemon meringue pie (see page 88)

WEDNESDAY
Breakfast
½ grapefruit
1 fried egg
25g/1oz grilled lean bacon
15g/½ oz fried bread

Lunch
100g/4oz grilled plaice
50g/2oz chips
100g/4oz green beans
1 tablespoon tomato ketchup
1 apple or pear

Dinner
2 egg omelette
50g/2oz mushrooms, grilled with little fat
lettuce, cucumber, tomato
15g/½ oz bread with 7g/¼ oz butter or 15g/½ oz low-fat spread
1 banana or 2 apples

THURSDAY
Breakfast
½ grapefruit
1 boiled egg

Lunch
small glass unsweetened orange juice
2 beefburgers
2 tomatoes
100g/4oz grilled mushrooms
1 fried egg
50g/2oz chips
1 tablespoon tomato ketchup

Dinner
½ grapefruit
100g/4oz grilled plaice
100g/4oz green beans
50g/2oz jacket potato
7g/¼oz butter or 15g/½oz low-fat spread
1 pear

FRIDAY
Breakfast
½ grapefruit
1 boiled egg
25g/1oz wholemeal bread
7g/¼oz butter

Lunch
100g/4oz roast lean beef
50g/2oz jacket potato
25g/1oz Yorkshire pudding
100g/4oz cabbage
100g/4oz green beans
little thin gravy
100g/4oz stewed apple
1 tablespoon whipped cream

Dinner
1 egg omelette
Winter salad (see page 86)
1 pear
1 orange

SATURDAY
Breakfast
½ grapefruit
1 egg omelette or 1 scrambled egg

Lunch
50g/2oz wholemeal bread
15g/½ oz butter
1 tomato, lettuce leaf, 2 slices cucumber
1 teaspoon salad cream
7g/¼ oz grated hard cheese
(all above ingredients made into a sandwich)
1 apple or orange

Dinner
100g/4oz melon weighed with skin
1 large grilled lean lamb chop or 100g/4oz roast lean meat
75g/3oz carrots
100g/4oz cabbage
glass of dry sherry
1 apple

SUNDAY
Breakfast
1 egg, scrambled, poached or boiled
25g/1oz toast
1 tomato, if liked

Lunch
3 fish fingers, grilled
75g/3oz peas
50g/2oz chips
100g/4oz fresh fruit salad (no sugar)

Dinner
clear soup
100g/4oz lean steak
50g/2oz jacket potato
100g/4oz green beans
1 tomato
1 apple

Diet No 4   1,200-Calorie Diet (No 2/Women)

I designed this diet for a one-week sponsored slim which I
organised in aid of local charities. The weight losses
experienced were excellent – with the maximum weight loss
during the week being 10 pounds (4.5 kilos) and 4-5 pounds
(1.75-2.25 kilos) being average. These weight losses were
experienced by women who had been dieting for some time
and had lost substantial amounts of weight prior to the slim,
again confirming my conviction that we don't need to starve
to lose weight.

The style of this diet allows maximum freedom of choice
and versatility – my slimmers loved it!

You are allowed three meals a day. In addition to these,
you are allowed 150 calories which may be used as you wish.
The meals may be eaten at any time.

To be consumed daily
300ml/ ½ pint fresh milk *or* 600ml/1 pint skimmed milk
15g/ ½ oz butter or margarine *or* 25g/1oz low-fat spread
Tea and coffee may be drunk freely, provided that your milk
allowance is not exceeded and that artificial sweeteners are
used in place of sugar. Low-calorie squashes, slimline
drinks, pure lemon juice and water are also unrestricted.

Breakfasts
1 ½ fresh grapefruit, 1 boiled or poached egg, 25g/1oz
   bread, butter from allowance.
2 ½ fresh grapefruit, 25g/1oz grilled lean bacon, 100g/4oz
   tomatoes, 25g/1oz bread, 15g/ ½ oz marmalade, butter
   from allowance.
3 90ml/3 fl oz unsweetened orange juice, 15g/ ½ oz Corn-

flakes or similar cereal, 150ml/¼ pint milk (additional to allowance), 1 teaspoon sugar.

4   ½ fresh grapefruit, 1 Weetabix or Shredded Wheat or 3 tablespoons All Bran, 150ml/¼ pint milk (additional to allowance), 2 teaspoons sugar.

Main Meals

1   175ml/6oz clear or low calorie soup. 75g/3oz lean red meat or 100g/4oz chicken or 225g/8oz steamed white fish, 100g/4oz green leafy vegetables, 100g/4oz carrots, 50g/2oz potato (new or jacket), little thin gravy (Oxo or similar) if desired. 100g/4oz stewed fruit (no sugar).

2   Large salad comprising lettuce, tomatoes, cucumber, celery, spring onions, grated raw carrot, ½ hard-boiled egg, and 50g/2oz cold lean meat or 75g/3oz chicken or 25g/1oz hard cheese (eg. Cheddar) or 100g/4oz cottage cheese. 25g/1oz low-calorie salad dressing. 75g/3oz jacket potato or 25g/1oz bread (butter from allowance). 100g/4oz stewed fruit (no sugar) or baked apple.

3   175ml/6 fl oz clear or low calorie soup. 50g/2oz liver, 25g/1oz grilled lean bacon, 2 tomatoes, 50g/2oz thick-cut chips, 100g/4oz green beans. 100g/4oz fresh fruit salad.

4   1 large sausage, 1 fried egg, 50g/2oz thick-cut chips, 2 grilled tomatoes, 100g/4oz green leafy vegetables, 100g/4oz carrots. 25g/1oz ice cream.

5   Two egg omelette with 15g/½ oz hard cheese and 50g/2oz grilled mushrooms, large salad, 100g/4oz jacket potato or 50g/2oz thick-cut chips. 1 small pear.

Snack Meals

1   25g/1oz toast with 15g/½ oz hard cheese and 1 poached egg, garnished with 1 sliced tomato.

2   50g/2oz bread made into a sandwich with lettuce, cucumber, tomato, 2 slices hard-boiled egg, 15g/½ oz grated cheese. Use a little low-calorie salad dressing if desired.

3   1 fried egg, 50g/2oz thick-cut chips, 50g/2oz peas.

4   2 cream crackers or crispbreads, 15g/½ oz hard cheese, 150g/5oz carton fruit yoghurt or 2 pieces fresh fruit.

5   2 hard-boiled eggs with salad, 1 crispbread (butter from allowance).
6   100g/4oz cottage cheese (with or without chives or pineapple) on 2 crispbreads (butter from allowance).
7   1 small tin of one of the following: spaghetti bolognaise, spaghetti in tomato and cheese sauce, spaghetti hoops, ravioli or baked beans, plus 25g/1oz toast.

You may have one 'treat' per day amounting to approximately 150 calories. A few suggestions are as follows:

small packet crisps
150g/5oz carton flavoured yoghurt
extra 300ml/ ½ pint fresh milk
2 tablespoons double cream
25g/1oz sweets
1 doughnut
65g/2 ½ oz ice cream
1 small cake
2 chocolate digestive biscuits
300ml/ ½ pint beer
2 whiskies or other spirits
25g/1oz chocolate
3 plain biscuits

In fact, you may choose anything providing the calorie value does not exceed 150. If in doubt as to calorie values buy a calorie book from your local bookshop, or check the chart at the end of this book.

Each day select one breakfast, one main meal, one snack meal (from the above diet-plan) and a 'treat' of your choice. Breakfast should be eaten before 10.30 am – and try to eat *slowly*.

Diet No 5   1,000-Calorie Diet

Only attempt this diet if you have lost weight on a higher calorie intake diet previously but have now reached another plateau, and are within a few pounds (or kilos) of achieving your desired weight. Choose four meals from the lists, selecting one meal from each of the various sections. For maximum results, each meal should be eaten at least two hours before the next one. However, for convenience it may be preferable to combine two on occasions.

If you have hopes of eating normally again, it is most important that you do not remain on this diet for longer than four weeks. Should your weight reach a plateau at this stage, you should *increase* your calorie intake to 1,200 for four weeks. This may be achieved either by resorting to one of the 1,200 calorie diets or by consuming one extra meal from this diet. During this time you may even lose a little weight, but the main purpose of the exercise is to increase your level of eating so that a drop to 1,000 calories will effect a significant weight loss again. This really is very effective – so please be patient.

Each day select one meal from each section, ie. breakfast, main meal and snack meal plus two items from the fruit section. You are also allowed a treat amounting to 70 calories per day.

To be consumed daily
300ml/½ pint fresh milk (or 600ml/1 pint skimmed milk)
7g/¼ oz butter or margarine (or 15g/½ oz low-fat spread).

Breakfasts

1 15g/½ oz (dry weight) oatmeal made into porridge with water, served with 120ml/4oz milk additional to allowance and 1 teaspoon sugar.
2 ½ fresh grapefruit, 1 boiled egg, 1 crispbread.
3 ½ fresh grapefruit, 25g/1oz grilled lean bacon, tomatoes.
4 1 small egg, 25g/1oz toast.
5 ½ fresh grapefruit, 15g/½ oz cheese on 25g/1oz toast, 1 tomato.
6 1 Shredded Wheat or 1 Weetabix, 120ml/4oz milk additional to allowance, 1 teaspoon sugar.
7 15g/½ oz Cornflakes, Special K, Frosties, All-Bran or similar cereal, 120ml/4fl oz milk additional to allowance, 1 teaspoon sugar.

Main Meals

1 50g/2oz lean red meat or 75g/3oz poultry, 100g/4oz cauliflower or cabbage or similar green vegetable, plus 100g/4oz carrots and 25g/1oz potato. Thin gravy if desired.

2 Large salad with ½ hard-boiled egg plus 25g/1oz hard cheese or 100g/4oz cottage cheese or 50g/2oz lean meat (ham, pork, etc.), 25g/1oz low-calorie dressing. Stewed rhubarb (no sugar).

3 2 egg omelette filled with grilled mushrooms and tomatoes, served with green salad.

4 3 grilled fish fingers, 100g/4oz sliced green beans, 100g/4oz carrots, 15g/½oz low-calorie tartare sauce or 25g/1oz tomato ketchup.

5 50g/2oz grilled liver, 25g/1oz grilled lean bacon, 1 grilled onion, 100g/4oz carrots, 100g/4oz cauliflower or similar. Tomato.

6 175g/6oz steamed white fish (cod, plaice, haddock, etc.), 50g/2oz new potatoes, 100g/4oz sliced green beans, 100g/4oz carrots, 25g/1oz tomato ketchup or 15g/½oz low-calorie tartare sauce.

7 1 egg fried in non-stick pan, 75g/3oz thick-cut chips, 50g/2oz peas, grilled tomatoes.

8 100g/4oz canned salmon, 75g/3oz peas, 50g/2oz potatoes.

9 50g/2oz ham, 1 ring fresh pineapple, 50g/2oz peas, 50g/2oz new potatoes, 2 tomatoes.

Snack Meals

1 25g/1oz bread with 15g/½oz Edam cheese and 1 poached egg. Garnish with 1 sliced tomato.

2 Large salad with ½ hard-boiled egg and 25g/1oz Edam cheese or 40g/1½oz lean meat. 25g/1oz low-calorie salad dressing.

3 3 starch reduced rolls filled with lettuce, tomatoes, cucumber, onion, ½ hard-boiled egg and 15g/½oz grated cheese. Spread with a scraping of low-fat spread and 15g/½oz low-calorie salad dressing.

4 1 large apple, 50g/2oz Edam cheese or 40g/1½oz hard cheese, 1 tomato.

5 25g/1oz toast, 150g/5oz canned baked beans or spaghetti.

6 25g/1oz grilled lean bacon, 100g/4oz tinned or fresh tomatoes, 100g/4oz sliced green beans, 15g/½oz toast.

7 150g/5oz smoked haddock, 1 poached egg, 1 tomato, 100g/4oz sliced green beans.

8   50g/2oz bread made into sandwiches (or 1 large bread roll or cob) with one of the following fillings:
    (a) 15g/½ oz grated cheese
    (b) 1 size 6 small hard-boiled egg
    (c) 25g/1oz chicken
    (d) 25g/1oz lean ham
    (e) 40g/1½ oz salmon
    (f) 7g/¼ oz cheese, 2 slices hard-boiled egg, 1 teaspoon low-calorie salad dressing
    (g) 20g/¾ oz tongue
    (h) 20g/¾ oz luncheon meat
    (i) 20g/¾ oz corned beef
    (j) 20g/¾ oz roast lean beef

With each of these sandwich fillings you may add lettuce, cucumber and tomato if you wish, making a mammoth salad sandwich which will be very satisfying.

Fruit
Select any two of the following each day:

1 average apple	1 large grapefruit
1 average pear	75g/3oz grapes
1 average orange	75g/3oz banana (weighed
100g/4oz fresh fruit salad	without skin)
100g/4oz stewed fruit	1 large peach
(no sugar)	150g/5oz plums (fresh)

Snacks or Treats
Select only one per day:

1 can low-calorie soup
150g/5oz carton natural yoghurt
1 slice bread with butter from allowance made into a sandwich with 1 tomato
1 crispbread spread with yeast extract, plus 25g/1oz cottage cheese and 1 tomato
150ml/¼ pint milk additional to allowance
1 glass sherry
1 measure of any spirit
1 cream cracker plus 7g/¼ oz any cheese
1 plain digestive biscuit
1 wafer bar of vanilla ice cream

25g/1oz chips
25g/1oz sultanas
1 extra piece of fruit
15g/½ oz chocolate
1 packet of Polos
1 size 6 small egg
1 tablespoon double cream
20g/¾ oz sugar
75g/3oz boiled new potatoes
OR you may select another item not listed – but it must contain no more than 70 calories.

Diet No 6   The 'Eat-to-Live' type diet

The following is an easy-going diet which allows the slimmer to select favourite foods in quantities to satisfy the natural appetite. You may eat as much meat and fish as you wish, also eggs and Edam and cottage cheese. You are allowed a small amount of carbohydrate-rich food and unlimited quantities of most vegetables and fruit. The 'catch' is that certain foods are strictly forbidden – mostly those which contain large amounts of sugar, flour or fat.

This diet is ideal for people who cannot be bothered to count calories as the nature of the diet automatically restricts the calorie intake. It's also excellent for educating your appetite towards nutritional eating, because the 'forbidden foods' contain few nutrients. You will find no allowance for treats as in previous diets, but with such a vast list of 'free' foods from which to choose, I feel sure you will be able to satisfy any cravings without stepping outside the recommended guide lines.

Expectant mothers and children would be advised to use this diet because of the unlimited allowances of protein-rich foods. However, a word of warning before you eat a massive steak followed by 175g/6oz Edam cheese – for this diet to be effective you must eat *sensible* amounts of food. If you are a big eater, you may find results are very slow!

You may eat or drink as much as you like of the following:

Lean meat, poultry, rabbit, liver, kidney, heart, lean ham,

lean bacon, eggs, Edam and cottage cheese, fish of all kinds.

Fruit: (fresh or frozen or stewed without sugar) blackberries, gooseberries, melon, lemon, blackcurrants, grapefruit, raspberries, rhubarb, cherries, loganberries, redcurrants, strawberries.

Vegetables: asparagus, artichokes, beans (French or runner), broccoli, Brussels sprouts, Brussel tops, cabbage, carrots, cauliflower, celery, cucumber, chicory, endive, leeks, lettuce, marrow, mushrooms, mustard-cress, onions, spring onions, peppers, radishes, spinach, spring greens, swedes, tomatoes, turnips and watercress.

Drinks and Seasonings etc: Tea, coffee (using milk from allowance), water, soda water, low-calorie fruit squashes, tomato juice, slimmers' minerals. Oxo, Bovril, Marmite, broth, home-made vegetable soups, herbs, spices, flavouring, gelatine for sweet and savoury jellies, vinegar pickles, salt, pepper, mustard, vinegar.

YOU MUST EAT NOTHING ELSE WHATEVER EXCEPT YOUR DAILY ALLOWANCE.

Each day consume not more than:
300ml/ ½ pint fresh milk
15g/ ½ oz butter or any kind of fat
3 thin slices of wholemeal bread*
2 pieces of fresh fruit**
25g/1oz cheese

One slice of bread can be exchanged for one of the following:
2 cream crackers
1 ½ crispbreads
1 potato (size of an egg)
1 small helping of Yorkshire pudding
1 small helping of breakfast cereal
15g/ ½ oz (dry weight) rice or spaghetti

**1 piece of fresh fruit is:*
1 medium apple, 1 medium peach,
1 medium orange, 1 small banana,
1 medium pear or 10 medium grapes

Nuts and sausages may *sometimes* be exchanged for meat, fish or eggs.

Average helpings of the following *vegetables* may be exchanged for bread: beans (baked, broad, butter or haricot), beetroot, parsnips, peas.

Methods of cooking: NO FRYING, but you may bake, braise, poach, steam, boil, grill or roast (using no fat). Use an artificial sweetener for sweetening.

SUGGESTED MENU

Breakfast
½ grapefruit (optional)
1 egg or lean bacon and grilled tomatoes OR average helping
    grilled or poached fish, 1 slice bread
Cup of tea or coffee

Lunch
average helping of lean meat, poultry, offal or fish, 2 helpings
    of vegetables
fruit

Dinner
clear soup
average helping of meat, fish, eggs or cheese
salad or vegetables
1 slice bread or 1 small potato
fruit

Drinks may be taken between meals. Lunch and Dinner menus are interchangeable.

FORBIDDEN FOODS
Sugar, sorbitol, jam, marmalade, honey, treacle, golden
    syrup, lemon curd, peanut butter, glucose, diabetic jam.
Sweets of all kinds, chocolates, diabetic chocolate.
Cakes, buns, biscuits, pastries, tarts, puddings, flour.
Fats: cream, evaporated milk, cream cheese, ice cream, salad
    cream or mayonnaise, crisps or chips.
Fruit: canned and dried fruits.

Drinks: alcohol, fizzy drinks, fruit squashes, Ribena, Lucozade, lemonade, Bournvita, Horlicks, Ovaltine, cocoa, drinking chocolate, bottle coffee.

Pickles: sweet pickles.

Sauces: white sauce and all other sauces based on white sauce, eg. cheese or parsley sauce. Sweet sauces and custard. Very thick gravies; canned or packet soups.

For this diet to be effective, you MUST avoid these forbidden foods and drinks.

4

A Diet Plan for Hopeless Cases

After many attempts at various ways of dieting I found this method of calorie control to be invaluable. It requires time and patience but if you genuinely wish to lose those excess pounds (or kilos), you will *find* the time. Basically, the idea is that instead of thinking about a day's food allowance, you think in terms of a full week's. With the week's total calorie allowance in mind, you prepare a list of your favourite foods from which you just cross off each item as you eat it. There are three major benefits with this foolproof plan:

1 It means that you select only the foods you like, as and when you fancy them, thus avoiding the need for between-meal cheats.
2 By allowing yourself a certain amount of freedom, you gradually learn to eat sensibly, satisfying only your *natural* appetite.
3 If you want to over-eat one day, you can do so with a clear conscience because you just cross similar items off the list of foods as you eat them. You will soon realise that if you over-eat today there will be less food to last you for the rest of the week – so it won't be long before you realise the folly of being greedy!

First of all, prepare a list of your favourite foods together with calorie values per ounce (or gram) or per item, eg. 25g/1oz Cheddar Cheese = 120 calories, 1 Mars Bar = 300. And it's essential for you to divide your list into the various nutritional sections.

Include a 'treats' section where you list the foods or drinks for which you feel a great desire! Ironically, the food we

crave is often of little nutritional value – but a small treat can
be the key to the success of a diet.

My *own* short list looks like this:

My Personal Calorie Chart
(Calorie values given here are rounded up or down to the
nearest unit of 5, enabling easier calculation.)

	Calories per 25g/1oz		Calories per 25g/1oz
Bread and Cereals		Bananas	20
Bread, 1 thin slice from large		Grapefruit	5
loaf	70	Grapes	15
Breakfast cereals (average)	110	Melon	5
Crispbreads each	25	Orange	10
Rice, boiled	50	Orange juice (unsweetened)	10
Weetabix (1 biscuit)	55	Pears	10
Cheese		Tomatoes	5
Cheddar	120	*Meat*	
Cottage cheese	30	Bacon, lean, grilled	100
Double Gloucester	105	Beef, raw	50
Dutch Edam	85	roast	65
Dairy foods		minced with fat	
Butter	210	drained	60
Cream, single	60	Chicken, roast	50
whipping	100	Corned beef	65
Ice cream	60	Ham, lean	60
Lard	255	Lamb, roast	70
Low-fat spread	105	Liver	50
Milk (silver top)		Pork, roast, lean	90
600ml/1 pint	370	*Miscellaneous*	
Eggs		Gravy (thin) per tablespoon	5
1 boiled or poached	90	Jelly (¼ packet made with	
1 fried	135	water)	80
Fish (raw)		Low-calorie salad dressing	50
Cod	25	Low-calorie tartare sauce	50
Haddock	30	Soup, thin, home made or	
Plaice	20	low-calorie brand,	
Fruit		approx	5
Apples	10	Tomato ketchup	30

	Calories per 25g/1oz		Calories per 25g/1oz
*Treats		cauliflower, asparagus, green sliced beans, broccoli, onions	5
1 Choc ice	135		
Chocolate	160	Chips, thick, straight cut	40
1 chocolate digestive biscuit	130	crinkle cut	75
1 Mars bar	300	Crisps	150
1 packet Polos	90	Leeks	10
1 slice cake, between	200-400	Mushrooms, grilled	5
1 slice Slimmer's gâteau	130	fried	50
Sweets, approx	150	Peas	20
Vegetables		Potatoes, boiled or jacket	25
Baked beans	20	Salad (for one serving) to include lettuce, cucumber, cress, celery, onions	25
Brussels sprouts, bean sprouts	10		
Carrots, cabbage,			

*These have very little nutritional value.

It is vital that your diet contains sufficient quantities of the essential nutrients, so let's discuss your protein allowance first.

As protein helps to keep you feeling satisfied for longer, it is recommended that you should eat some form of meat, fish, eggs or cheese at each meal (including breakfast). Think ahead to what you will be eating at mid-day and list the meat and fish portions accordingly. Likewise, list the protein-rich foods to be included in your evening meals. Endeavour to include one meal per week of liver or kidneys to ensure an adequate supply of iron.

Many people find 300ml/½ pint fresh milk adequate to meet a day's tea and coffee requirements. I find that if I allow myself 600ml/1 pint milk, I can have as many drinks as I require – and this helps prevent me cheating!

Rather than working out exactly which vegetables you will eat at any particular meal, allow yourself a number of ounces (grams) of vegetables which contain only 5 calories per 1oz(25g). You are then free to choose between carrots, broccoli, sliced green beans, cabbage, cauliflower, celery, spinach, asparagus, etc. If you like peas, list them separately.

With regard to fruits, remember to allow yourself at least two helpings daily, as with the vegetables.

If you like sandwiches for your lunch, calculate your daily requirement and multiply by seven and add it to your list. The same applies with potatoes, rice, pasta, etc. Don't be frightened to include what you would *like* to eat. You can always reduce the quantities if, when you come to add up the list, the total is far too great a number of calories.

If you allow yourself 14 slices of bread for the week, you will probably want a reasonable quantity of butter to spread on it. If you don't object to the low-calorie spreads, you would be well advised to use these instead of butter as they work out at less than half the number of calories. Weigh out the week's butter allowance and keep it in a separate dish labelled accordingly! You could have two containers, one containing butter and the other containing low-fat spread for use in sandwiches.

You may now commence your list of foods required for seven days' eating. Remember to calculate the total calories accordingly. However, your list must contain the following:

14-21 portions of protein-rich foods
2 litres/3 ½ pints milk
14 (approx.) portions of carbohydrate foods
14 + portions vegetables (100g/4oz per portion)
14 + pieces of fresh fruit
100g/4oz butter or similar fat or 200g/7oz low-fat spread

A typical list might read as follows – but notice that next to items where there is a multiple allowance (eg. 6 eggs) each egg is indicated by a figure '1', so that each one may be crossed off after it has been eaten.

Total Food Allowance for One Week

Food	Units			Total Calories
6 rashers (100g/4oz) bacon	1 1 1 1 1 1			400
Chicken (3 portions)	100g/4oz	100g/4oz	100g/4oz	600
1 packet frozen braised beef				90

Food	Units	Total Calories
Liver	100g/4oz	200
Minced beef	100g/4oz	240
Steamed plaice	175g/6oz	120
6 eggs (boiled or poached)	1 1 1 1 1 1	540
175g/6oz Dutch Edam cheese (6 portions)	1 1 1 1 1 1	510
100g/4oz lean ham (2 portions)	50g/2oz 50g/2oz	240
600ml/1 pint fresh milk daily		2,590
100g/4oz butter		840
175g/6oz bread (6 slices)	1 1 1 1 1 1	420
350g/14oz potatoes (new) 100g/4oz 100g/4oz 50g/2oz 50g/2oz 50g/2oz		280
100g/4oz thick-cut chips (2 portions)	50g/2oz 50g/2oz	160
Soup: 1 tin low-calorie		60
Vegetables: 21 × 100g/4oz portions = 3 helpings per day (5 calories per 25g/1oz) 100g/4oz		420
100g/4oz peas (2 portions)	50g/2oz 50g/2oz	80
Fruit: 8 apples	1 1 1 1 1 1 1 1	320
4 oranges	1 1 1 1	200
4 grapefruits	½ ½ ½ ½ ½ ½ ½ ½	120
2 bananas	1 1	160
200g/8oz grapes (4 portions) 50g/2oz 50g/2oz 50g/2oz 50g/2oz		120
3 pears	1 1 1	120
3 salads (excluding tomatoes)	1 1 1	75
1.25kg/3lb tomatoes (25) 50g/2oz		250
100g/4oz low-calorie salad dressing (4 servings)	1 1 1 1	200
25g/1oz low-calorie tartare sauce	1	50

7/ 9,405

1,344

As I allow myself 1,500 calories per day, a residue of nearly 160 enables me to enjoy a daily treat – or I can save them up!

After making out your list, you must add together all the calories contained therein. Then divide the total by seven to give you your average daily intake. If this figure is too high, look again at the foods you have listed and see if you can trim down quantities.

The ideal is for your list to leave you with sufficient calories to allow yourself a treat. These extra calories can really help with regard to the occasional social drink – or the friend who says, 'you must have a piece of my super new cake – it cost me a fortune to make with all that brandy and cream in it!'

Cross off each item as you place it on your plate – and if you should happen to eat something that is not listed (for instance, if you were suddenly asked out for a meal), when you return home cross off similar 'types' of food from your list. It is important that you do not cross out a protein portion in exchange for a slice of gâteau! Your gâteau must be exchanged for a carbohydrate food or taken as three days' treats!

I am sure you will find this way of dieting fun, and it's super to be able to look at your list and think: 'What shall I have today – there's all this food to choose from, and it's all for me to eat as and when I want it.'

At this point I would suggest that after the fourth day you make a list of the foods remaining so that you can plan, to some degree, the remaining three days' menus.

So often when we're dieting we go off the rails and eat loads of foods we know we shouldn't be eating – and then resign ourselves to the fact that we've 'failed yet again'. With this type of diet, 'sins' can be immediately deducted from the weekly allowance and I found myself stopping an eating binge much earlier, realising that no damage was done if I stopped after the first illegal nibble. It isn't that *first* chocolate biscuit that puts the weight back on, you know – it's the second, third, fourth, fifth, sixth . . . that does it!

5

Easy Slimming

One of the most effective ways of dieting is to modify your existing eating pattern, retaining the basic meal-pattern but reducing the quantities of some foods and substituting low-calorie foods wherever possible.

The first experience I had of this was when my father complained that he had gained about 1½ stones (9.5 kilos) since retiring a few years earlier, and asked if I could design a diet specially for him. He detailed an average day's eating pattern and it read as follows:

Time	Food	Cups of tea*
6 am	Porridge, honey and cream	2
8 am	2 slices buttered toast and marmalade	2
11 am	Piece of cake	2
12.30 pm	Meat and vegetables, ice cream	2
4.30 pm	1 slice toast with cheese	2
7.30 pm	Biscuits	2
9.30 pm	Large serving of soup	–

*All sweetened with artificial sweetener.

I didn't consider it necessary to calculate the calorie intake because I knew that by making a few adjustments here and there, whatever the total was originally, the modified diet that I would recommend would be significantly lower in calories. It would therefore automatically effect an acceptable weight loss.

One factor which I did consider important was the knowledge that my father enjoyed his food very much – and any diet which left him with a single hunger pang would be doomed to failure! Also, he obviously enjoyed eating many meals in a day – far more than most people.

I suggested the following:

6 am	Porridge made with water, honey and top of the milk.
8 am	Small glass unsweetened orange or grapefruit juice. 1 boiled egg, 25g/1oz toast lightly spread with low-fat spread.
11 am	2 crispbreads lightly spread with low-fat spread and Marmite, 1 tomato.
12.30 pm	Lean meat and plenty of vegetables – but 1 potato only. (Grill meat where possible.) Ice cream – 1 scoop only.
4.30 pm	25g/1oz toast with 40g/1½oz cheese and a little low-fat spread, or a salad. Piece of fresh fruit.
7.30 pm	1 crispbread with Marmite and low-fat spread.
9.30 pm	Large serving of low-calorie soup.

The quantity of fluid was unrestricted, but a daily ration of 450ml/¾ pint fresh milk was recommended and obviously the habit of using artificial sweeteners in cups of tea should be continued.

Father was surprised to see that he could still eat his numerous meals – and was amazed to find he was actually eating *more* food, but fewer calories. In two and a half months he had lost a stone (6 kilos) and he has continued to follow the general pattern of this new diet – though now he enjoys an extra slice of cake when he fancies it!

As I explained in an earlier chapter, a diet should fit into *your* way of life so that it doesn't become a nuisance. In fact I believe you should *enjoy* your diet – my father did and still does!

Here are a few hints which might help you trim down the calories, but not the quantities, of *your* everyday eating pattern.

Breakfasts

'I like cereals because I can't face anything cooked.'

Did you know that one Weetabix is only 57 calories? As well as being low in calories, it is also very nutritious. If you

57

suffer from constipation, Bran Buds contain only 69 calories per 25g/1oz so may certainly be included in your diet. Skimmed milk on your cereal, with liquid artificial sweetener added, will reduce your calories even further at breakfast time.

'I like a cooked breakfast.'

Boiled or poached, a large (size 1, 2 or 3) egg works out at around 90 calories. Fry it and it jumps up to about 135 calories! If you possess a non-stick frying pan you can dry-fry, saving those 45 unwanted calories. But if not, wipe round your frying pan with a butter or lard wrapping paper and cook your egg slowly, covering it with a lid. This will ensure that your egg cooks completely – but it will absorb virtually no fat.

Scrambled egg is often given a high calorie value because butter is added during cooking – this way, one egg scrambled could total as much as 200 calories and that's before you even think about placing it on a slice of buttered toast (150 calories)! If you like your egg scrambled, warm a little milk (with salt and pepper added) in a saucepan. Stir in your egg and cook slowly. Calorie value is around 100, 1 slice of toast 70 calories, scraping of low-fat spread 30 calories, total 200.

If you like bacon or sausages, always grill them – because all that fat dripping into the grill pan is *saving* you 226 calories per 25g/1oz. And don't be tempted to dip your bread in it! (Remember to grill meat whenever you possibly can, as it is one of the easiest ways of cutting calories.)

If you must have fried bread, scrape half a slice of bread with a little lard or dripping on both sides and then grill it. This saves you lots of calories yet still looks and tastes like its calorie-soaked brother!

One of my favourite breakfasts is grilled bacon with grilled tomatoes. The total calories for one back rasher and 100g/4oz tomatoes is only about 85, yet I feel that I have started the day really well.

'I can't face any more than just toast for breakfast.'

If you can't manage anything more nutritious, toast is certainly better than nothing and wholemeal bread is to be recommended because it is more nutritious and satisfies you for longer. If proper wholemeal bread is difficult to find in your area, then sliced white bread is to be recommended rather than unsliced as I feel few dieters could be trusted to cut a thin, 25g/1oz slice every time!

Slimming breads can be very useful – but remember that the slices are quite small so you might be tempted to have more than one! Two slices of light bread contain as many calories as a thin slice off a large ordinary loaf.

As to what to spread on to your toast, the low-fat spreads can save you lots of calories. But they contain a proportion of water in their ingredients and can make hot toast go rather soggy – so either eat it quickly or spread it when the toast is cool. There is available an excellent low-calorie marmalade to spread on your toast. Alternatively, you could just scrape on a little ordinary marmalade.

Fruit is quite acceptable at breakfast time, particularly grapefruit. Half a large grapefruit has only 15 calories and will supply a valuable amount of your daily Vitamin C requirement. Try to have one every day, irrespective of whatever other food you eat at breakfast.

'I honestly can't face anything for breakfast – but I do get hungry mid-morning.'
If you haven't eaten any breakfast, be sure to eat something reasonably nutritious mid-morning. An apple and a small piece of cheese is much better than a chocolate bar. Two crispbreads spread with low-fat spread and Marmite provide a good mid-morning snack, or try a 150g/5oz carton of yoghurt.

If you have had breakfast but feel you need something to eat with your mid-morning cup of coffee, have a plain biscuit. Just one – and put the tin back on the top shelf *before* you eat it! Take your coffee and biscuit into another room to enjoy it!

Lunches
'I never know what to get for lunch because I'm on my own during the day and it doesn't seem worth cooking just for me.'
A salad can be very useful to the dieter as it is filling,

nutritious and provides roughage. It's unfortunate that dieting and 'rabbit food' are synonymous in the mind's eye of slimming cynics. A salad offering variety, well presented and served with a tasty dressing can be absolutely delicious. In my opinion low-calorie salad dressing is every bit as good as ordinary salad cream – and, at only 50 calories per 25g/1oz, can certainly be included in your salad.

A salad with a difference could be made by grating raw carrot, raw beetroot (it really does taste very good), bean sprouts, a little chopped lettuce, a few nuts and raisins, a slice or two of tomato, cucumber, hard-boiled egg, chopped onion and, instead of the usual dressing, try soy sauce. It is low in calories and very tasty.

Many slimmers believe that sandwiches are automatically banned from a diet. I believe that they should not be excluded if you enjoy eating your snack meal in sandwich form. But spread your bread with butter or low-calorie spread and then scrape it off again – ensuring that an absolute minimum remains! Alternatively, butter only one slice. Fill your sandwiches with lots of low-calorie goodies such as lettuce, tomato, cucumber – but include a slice of cheese or ham or a few slices of hard-boiled egg, then top with a little low-calorie salad dressing and there you will have a really substantial sandwich which will satisfy even the greediest of appetites! If you are feeling really strong-willed, you could fill starch-reduced rolls in the same way.

If you fancy an egg on toast for your lunch, sprinkle grated cheese on to the toast and put it under the grill before placing your poached egg on it. You will find this takes up fewer calories than butter and yet makes it more tasty. Garnish with a grilled tomato to complete your dish.

For cooked snack meals see page 44, where many suggested meal ideas are given.

Dinners

Many dieters believe that potatoes are real 'baddies', but they contain useful nutrients and are not very high in calories unless they are cooked in fat. If you adore chips, it's important to realise that straight, thick-cut chips amount to around 40 calories per 25g/1oz compared with thin crinkle-cut ones, which score an alarming 75 calories. Jacket potatoes are excellent for the slimmer as the skin provides extra roughage – and if you mash your old potatoes, use only milk, salt and pepper. No butter!

New potatoes contain only 21 calories per 25g/1oz. If I have a new potato or two on my dinner plate I feel I have had the same as everyone else and, psychologically, that helps me to accept my diet and eat in moderation. If I don't have any on my plate at the dinner table and there are a few left over after the meal, guess who eats them while carrying them out to the kitchen! Unfortunately, that small cheat is very often instrumental in causing a total diet breakdown for the remainder of that day.

I like to complete a meal with something sweet and there are plenty of lovely foods to eat without using up loads of calories. Ice cream, at 60 calories per 25g/1oz, is a good standby, and fruit made into a fresh fruit salad is always popular. Strawberries when they are in season are super for the slimmer at only 80 calories per 450g/1lb! And if you must have cream with them, use the 'top' of the milk from your daily allowance.

Rhubarb, at 2 calories per 25g/1oz, is a great friend of the slimmer. Cooked in a little water with artificial sweeteners added, it provides a delicious sweet or between-meal snack for the peckish dieter. Avoid eating vast amounts, though, as it's very acid.

Apples baked in their skins, cored and filled with a few sultanas, provide a delightful hot sweet. If they need any additional sweetener, add artificial sweetener in tablet or liquid form with the sultanas.

Later in this book you will find various recipes which I hope will be helpful. Believe it or not there is a recipe for 'Slimmer's Gâteau' (see page 88) which is absolutely delicious.

General hints on calorie saving when cooking

Remember that *fat* – and that means butter, margarine, cooking oil, lard etc. – is the highest calorie food that we consume. Use as little of it as possible but do not exclude it completely from your diet as butter, margarine and low-fat spreads contain some vitamins, and a little fat is essential.

Grill food whenever possible, as this can reduce calorie values of meats quite considerably.

Use artificial sweeteners to replace sugar whenever possible. It's a good idea to use a 'high class' sweetener for drinks but ordinary artificial sweetener tablets for cooking (available from any chemist at a considerably lower cost than branded lines). If you find artificial sweetener tablets too sweet, liquid sweetener may be the answer, as one drop equals ¼ teaspoon, or use ¼ teaspoon of the granulated sugar substitutes.

Many calories may be saved by using skimmed milk in place of fresh milk in the preparation of custard, sauces, table creams, Yorkshire puddings and so on.

I never buy double cream as I find 'whipping' cream thick enough for any purpose – and whipping cream costs less in money as well as in calories.

When making a jelly with canned fruit to be included, avoid using the syrup – at least not for your portion. Split the jelly in two and make it up as two separate 300ml/½ pints. Use water only in yours – and wash any canned fruit in order to remove the syrup. If your family are fortunate enough not to suffer from overweight, their jelly can be made up to include the syrup if you wish.

Of course, very low-calorie jellies can be made by using low-calorie orange or lemon or lime cordial, water and gelatine (see page 87). Add fresh fruit if desired.

Another useful tip is to do any preparation for the next meal immediately after the previous one. Foods like fruit salads can be prepared – and because I have just eaten my meal, I don't find myself consuming half the fruit as I prepare it! Having organised the next meal as far as possible, I then leave the kitchen until it is time to actually cook or serve it.

A slimming tip which I find most helpful is to use a smaller plate for meals. This automatically reduces the amount of food – but the fact that my plate is full is a positive psychological factor.

62

6

Binge Eating

One day I made a list of all that I had consumed during an eating binge, and it read thus:

1.00 pm   Cooked lunch of meat and vegetables, followed by strawberry mousse. Cup of coffee.

3.30 pm   Large helping of strawberry mousse.
Chocolate flake (large).
Cup of tea.
100g/4oz sultanas with 75g/3oz butter.
225g/8oz soft roes fried in butter with 50g/2oz boiled rice.
Packet of potato crisps.
3½ oz ice cream with cream and raspberry sauce.
More strawberry mousse.
2 bowls of cornflakes with top of milk and lots of sugar.
50g/2oz cheese.
Another chocolate flake.

It took me less than 1½ hours to consume the lot – and, as I ate each item, I was convinced that it would be the last. So the obvious question is *why*? Why did I eat all that food when I wasn't even hungry?

There is no obvious answer. Psychologists and psychiatrists offer interesting reasons for possible causes of these ridiculous outbursts of over-indulgence – but to my knowledge no one has yet produced the ultimate solution. For an analysis of binges and compulsive eating, see *Fat is a Feminist Issue* by Susie Orbach (Hamlyn Paperbacks).

It seems extraordinary that just when the desire to be slim seems to be the most important factor in our lives, we experience uncontrollable urges to gorge ourselves with high-calorie foods. And while it might take one or two months to lose a stone (6 kilos) – it could be gained again in a couple of weeks by someone who binged for several days.

And when the slimmer has a binge it is usually the high-calorie 'nonsense' foods that appeal, never the sensible, lower calorie types of food. It's as though we *want* to grow fat again.

Many slimmers, when they are binge eating, find themselves panicking as they continue to eat in vast quantities, possibly feeling that if they eat enough perhaps they will burst – or vomit. Some do. But when I was grossly overeating, I never vomited. I even tried to make myself do so, by sticking my fingers down my throat and drinking salt water, but to no avail. When that failed, I turned to laxatives, hoping that I might have more success in 'flushing all the food away' before it turned to fat! All the laxatives managed to do was give me dreadful stomach ache. No way did it succeed in preventing the excess food turning into fat. I must have been mad to do all those things – but no one knew that I was and therefore no one told me how utterly foolish I was being.

Whenever I over-ate drastically, I became very lethargic, even sleepy, and when I woke in the morning I felt dreadful. I had no energy, I was bad tempered and my stomach was still distended.

When we stop to think about the awful sensations experienced as a result of a binge, we must surely ask ourselves why we still do it. What good does it do us? What purpose does it serve?

I feel that many binges are caused by a slimmer sticking to a too-strict dieting regime, either in terms of the quantity or types of food allowed. For instance, people who are told not to eat any bread, cakes or biscuits will find infinite willpower for a limited period – but then, instead of having one slice of cake as a real treat, they may develop an instant, uncontroll-able craving for a whole cake!

The lesson to be learned here, I feel, is that eating plenty of food, including a little of what you fancy, within a generous calorie allowance suitable for you as an individual, is the *only* way to achieve long-term weight loss.

But we all occasionally feel a great desire to eat something outside our calorie allowance, often when we experience bad news or a disappointment. In these circumstances it's pointless to eat a small item (such as a very small chocolate bar) in an attempt to do the least amount of damage, calorie-wise, as it only leaves a craving for more. I have found that if I eat, for instance, a Mars bar (which I, personally, find infinitely satisfying), I do not crave for more. If I try to be economical, I find that I continue nibbling until the nibbling could be interpreted as a Henry VIII feast!

You must learn by your own experience and accept that occasionally you *will* cheat. Have your Mars bar or cream cake occasionally and that, on its own, will not make you gain weight while you are dieting. It is the mountains of food which you eat afterwards, because you feel you have failed on your diet, that do the damage. In actual figure terms the problem looks like this:

Average daily energy expenditure	2,000 calories
Calorie allowance during reducing campaign	1,400
Additional Mars bar	300
	1,700 calories.
	This still leaves a balance of 300 calories before reaching your daily requirement.

This illustrates how foolish it is to feel that your diet has totally collapsed just because you have eaten something extra.

If you feel your willpower is running thin at any time, try drinking a low-calorie fizzy drink. This acts as a wonderful filler for a hungry tum – and you'll probably find you won't eat as much as you would have done had you not had the drink. A couple of cups of tea or coffee (made with water) work just as well.

The next question to ask yourself is: what is it that you're craving for? Is it chocolate or cake or perhaps even egg and chips? Whatever it is – eat it now! And then busy yourself in some way immediately afterwards.

If you know you won't stop at one slice of cake, cut off one slice and, before you eat it, slice the remainder into the number of portions necessary to provide one slice for each member of the family. This avoids the temptation of repeatedly sneaking a tiny slice more. If, on the other hand, there is too much for your family, place some in your freezer if you have one, or ask a friend round for a cup of tea and offer her a slice. And you can always give the dog a treat, too! As long as he's not overweight, he can help you save yourself!

And there are other things you can do to avoid having a binge:

1 Occupy yourself in a dirty job such as weeding the garden or cleaning the oven. If your hands are dirty you won't want to bother to wash your hands every few minutes just to eat a biscuit!

2 If you know you are a biscuit/chocolate/cake nibbler, don't keep them in the house. If the family like them, they can buy their own, and they must lock them away out of your sight.

   One of my members gives the key to her freezer to her husband each morning to prevent her from eating lots of ice cream during the day! And this is a good way of keeping bread out of your way, too. Buy sliced loaves so that slices may be taken out frozen, as required, by another member of the family. Same with cakes and pastries!

3 Always keep a good stock of fresh fruit. It is money well spent to buy apples that look delicious and oranges that look really juicy – because you won't get fat by over-eating fruit.

4 When preparing food, always return *all* the remaining ingredients to their rightful storage positions, either in

the refrigerator or the pantry, before you eat. This helps to avoid unnecessary nibbling after a meal.

5 Try to prepare your next meal immediately after you complete the last one. You will not 'pick' so much as you will not be feeling hungry. I find this helps me tremendously.

But if you *have* had a binge, try this diet next day, but for *one day only*.

Binge Corrector Diet

Breakfast Whole grapefruit, cup of tea.
Lunch Steamed fish, green vegetable.
Dinner Clear soup, large salad with 1 hard-boiled egg and low-calorie dressing.
Supper Apple or pear, 1 plain biscuit.
Plus 150ml/¼ pint fresh milk in drinks.

7

Exercise

Exercise is good for everyone – assuming that they are sound in wind and limb – irrespective of whether or not they are dieting, but it is particularly helpful to the slimmer for two reasons. Firstly, it helps tone the body (encouraging a more attractive figure) and, secondly, it burns a few extra calories.

Exercise alone, however, will *not* make you lose weight. To use up sufficient extra energy to effect a weight loss, you would undoubtedly work up an enormous appetite! The answer, therefore, is to find a sensible form of exercise which appeals to you, and to combine it with a good slimming diet.

If you enjoy sport, then you will find that your weekly round of golf or game of squash or badminton will be ideal in encouraging a healthy, trim figure. If you are not a sporty type, jogging is a wonderful all-round toner. Remember to start off very slowly, gradually building up the distance and speed.

I personally feel that one of the best ways of toning every corner of your body is to practise Yoga regularly. It requires little energy, for it is the slow-motion movements and the holding of the extreme position of each posture which make Yoga unique and so beneficial. It also has a relaxing effect on both body and mind.

If you feel more energetic, you could try some keep-fit exercises. If you like pop music, it can be great fun working out your own routines in time to the music! Remember to start off every session with a warming-up period – and always relax for a few minutes at the end of your practise.

Here are some Yoga exercises which are particularly

helpful in toning the body while slimming.* Practise them as often as possible when you are on your own and able to enjoy peace and quiet. Avoid practising within 90 minutes after eating a meal – and remember that a few minutes a day is better than nothing. Follow the lettered diagrams.

Exercise 1: Deep Breathing

Stand upright, hands down by your sides, and exhale completely through your nose (**A**). (All Yoga deep breathing should be done through the nose, never the mouth.)

Begin breathing into the lower part of your lungs so that your abdomen distends (expands). Now allow your abdomen to pull in as you expand your chest and it fills with air, and finally fill the upper parts of your lungs (raise your shoulders if you wish). Hold the breath for a count of 3, then exhale slowly.

Repeat this exercise, counting to 9 as you inhale, hold for a count of 3 and exhale to the count of 9.

Now repeat this exercise again – but this time raise your arms above your head while inhaling as before (**B**).

Stretch your hands right up and stand on your toes while you hold the breath for a count of 3. Slowly exhale and lower your hands down to your sides.

Repeat this exercise twice more, breathing in and out through your nose at all times. Relax on completion by flopping forward from the hips and hanging your head and arms down in front of you. Let their weight draw you down.

Exercise 2: Waist Trimmer

Stand with your feet wide apart, hands and arms outstretched to your sides at shoulder level (**C**). Keeping your spine straight, slowly start bending sideways to the right. Arms go with you so that your right hand touches some part of your right leg and your left hand reaches over your head, as if trying to touch the wall to your right (**D**). Relax your head

*The exercises recommended will not injure or damage any healthy person, but responsibility cannot be accepted for any physical injury caused while following or obviously exceeding the recommended exercises. If in doubt, consult your doctor.

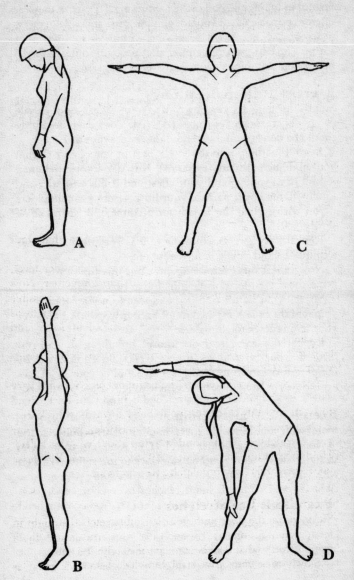

down to the right and hold this extreme position for a count of 15. Slowly return to the standing position, then pause for a moment and relax.

Repeat to the left side. Then repeat the whole routine once more.

Note It is important to keep the spine flat in this exercise. You may find a tendency to twist it forward slightly to enable you to reach further. However, the benefits to your waist are greater if you try to keep your spine flat.

Exercise 3: Backward and Forward Stretch

(Toning for the tummy, arms and legs – excellent for reducing midriff bulges!)

Stand in a good posture, with your feet comfortably together and your weight evenly distributed.

Raise your arms and bend your elbows so that your thumbs touch your chest (**E**).

Extend your arms out in front of you at shoulder level, then round to the back, clasping your hands together. Now extend your arms outwards and upwards as far as possible *without slumping forward* (**F**). Arms should be as straight as possible (this part of the exercise is excellent for round shoulders).

Begin to lean backwards, keeping your arms and hands extended (**G**), and hold for a count of 5.

Now slowly straighten up and begin to come forward very slowly, with hands still outstretched behind your back. Bend forward and down, taking your head towards your knees. Lean forward and down as far as possible, keeping your knees straight and your hands way up above your back (**H**). Hold the position for a count of 10. Slowly come up, release your arms and relax completely. Repeat twice more.

Exercise 4: Leg Stretches

Sit down on the floor with your legs outstretched straight in front of you. Sit up straight and raise your arms gracefully in front of you so that they become parallel with the floor.

Slowly raise your arms straight as you lean back as far as

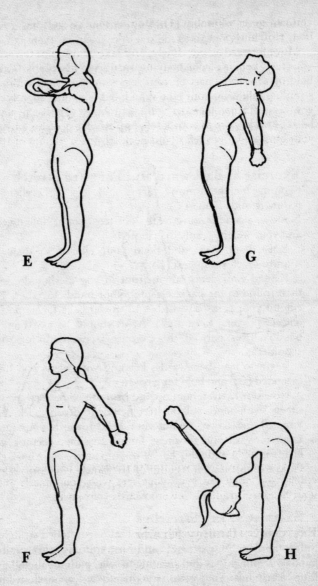

you can go comfortably **(I)**. Stop as soon as you feel your body stiffening or shaking.

Move forward again, slowly, and take your hands towards your feet, bending your body forward from your hips. Take hold of whichever part of your legs you can reach without straining, allowing your elbows to bend outwards slightly as you bend further forward with your body **(J)**. Keep your head down as close to your knees as possible, stretching from your hips, and try to relax your neck. Hold for a count of 10.

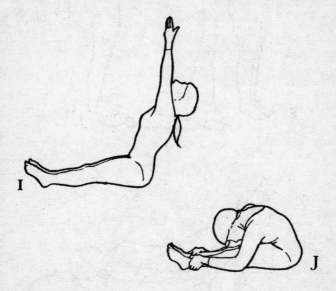

Repeat whole routine twice more.

As you progress, you will find that you will be able to hold either your ankles or even your feet with your hands and your head will gradually lower towards your knees.

Exercise 5: Tummy Firmer

Sit on the floor, legs straight out in front of you. Place your hands on your thighs and *slowly* lie down, giving yourself as little assistance as possible. As soon as your body is

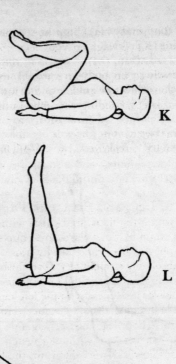

K

L

M

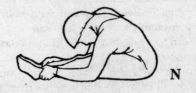

N

completely flat, slowly bend your knees and hold them close to your chest (**K**). Straighten your legs up into the air (**L**) and slowly lower them (**M**). As soon as they come to rest on the floor, slowly sit up and lean forward, touching your toes or holding your calves or ankles, and bring your head down towards your knees, bending your elbows slightly if you wish (**N**). Without pausing, begin to sit up again and repeat the whole routine twice more.

This exercise is particularly beneficial in toning all muscles in the abdomen and also in the legs and back. It should be performed in continuous slow motion.

Exercise 6: Legs and Buttocks Toner

Lie face down on the floor, make fists with your hands and place them, thumbs downward, by your sides (**O**). Place your chin on the floor and slowly raise your right leg, keeping it absolutely straight (**P**). (It is far better not to raise it too far but to keep it straight.) Hold for a count of 5 and then slowly lower it. Repeat with the left leg. Now raise both legs together (straight) a short distance. Hold for a count of 5. Finally, raise both legs together again – but this time as high as you can manage without causing any strain (**Q**). Hold for 5. Slowly lower them to the floor and relax completely.

Repeat whole routine once more.

Exercise 7: Toner for Front Thighs and Midriff Bulge

Kneel up, with your knees comfortably apart, about 12 inches (30cm) (**R**). Place your hands on your hips and *slowly* lean backwards as far as possible, curving your spine. Let your head go back as well (**S**), and then hold the extreme position for a count of 10.

Slowly return to a kneeling position and relax completely. Repeat once more.

As you progress you will be able to arch your back more and more and will enjoy greater benefits from this excellent posture. It helps to keep the spine supple and stretches the abdomen and thighs.

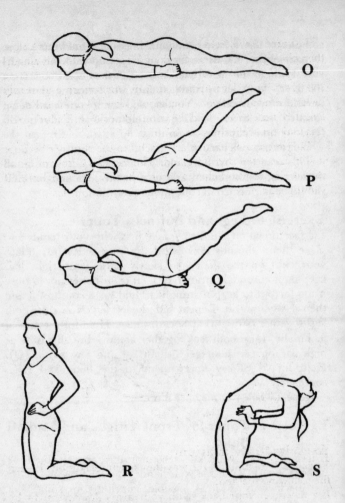

Exercise 8: Shoulder Stand

Loosen or remove anything that might constrict your neck
(zip, hair grip, etc.). Lie on your back on the floor and swing
your legs up into the air, supporting your back with your
hands (**T**). Aim to achieve as vertical a position as possible
with legs together. Hold for as long as is reasonably
comfortable (2-3 minutes if possible).

To come down from the shoulder stand, bend your knees, then place your hands on the floor for support. Slowly uncurl your spine so that your back becomes flat on the floor. Now straighten your legs up into the air once more and slowly lower them to the floor. You should now relax for the same length of time as you held the inverted position. Failure to do this may cause dizziness or fainting.

This exercise is particularly useful to the slimmer because it stimulates the thyroid gland. The increased flow of blood into the head also helps towards a healthy complexion and shining hair.

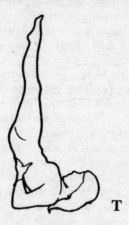

T

Exercise 9: Relaxation

Yoga teachers differ in the way they teach relaxation. I teach the following method:

Lie down on your back, with your arms down straight by your sides. Make sure that you are warm enough and comfortable. Place a pillow under your head, if necessary.

Concentrate first of all on your feet and tell yourself that they are becoming heavier and heavier and that they are sinking down and down into the floor. Just let them go – let them relax. This beautiful, relaxed feeling is creeping up your legs so that they, too, are beginning to feel heavy. First your calves, then your knees and then your thighs. All are feeling very, very heavy, sinking deeply into the floor. Allow them to relax completely.

Now concentrate on the lower abdomen – the pelvic muscles are beginning to relax and are feeling heavier and heavier, then your buttocks, your tummy and your spine – all are relaxing and getting heavier and heavier . . .

Now relax your chest and breathe very quietly as you let go of all the tensions you may hold in your chest and shoulders. Relax your chest completely.

The heavy feeling is creeping up and up and now your shoulders are completely relaxed. Your arms are beginning to feel heavy and are getting heavier and heavier. Your elbows, wrists and hands all feel very, very heavy and relaxed . . .

This beautiful feeling of relaxation is now reaching your neck and chin. Let them go; let them relax completely . . . The feeling reaches all parts of your face, your mouth, nose, cheeks, ears, eyes, forehead and scalp. Just let everything go completely and relax. Totally . . .

Your body becomes so relaxed that it feels like it is floating on a bed of fresh air. You feel as though you couldn't move a hand or foot if you wanted to . . .

Relax your mind by thinking beautiful, happy thoughts – spring flowers and sunshine; green fields and beautiful trees swaying in the breeze; lying in the warm sun on a beautiful secluded beach.

Let yourself go completely and relax totally . . .

When you feel ready, stretch all your limbs and sit up slowly, sitting still for a few moments while you 'wake up' completely.

After your Yoga practice you should feel revitalised but relaxed.

Further Reading

For more advice and guidance on doing Yoga, I can personally recommend Richard Hittleman's *Yoga for Health* (it has line drawings throughout), published by Hamlyn, and *Yoga for All Ages* by Rachel Carr (published by Collins).

8

Questions and Answers

Q. *'Why do I lose a lot of weight during the first week of dieting and then only lose about 2-3 pounds (1-1.5 kilos) thereafter, despite the fact that I eat the same number of calories each week? If occasionally I do over-eat I can gain as much as 4 pounds (1.75 kilos) in one evening. Why is this?'*

A. Most people enjoy a significant weight loss during the first week on a reducing diet. I remember one of our class members losing 16 pounds (7.25 kilos) during her first week of dieting! And while part of the loss shown on the scales is fat which has been burned up, there is usually a reduction primarily in the fluid level of the body during the first week of dieting, effected by the change in the type of food consumed.

Carbohydrate-rich foods tend to encourage fluid retention and, as soon as you embark on a reducing diet, the carbohydrate intake is likely to be reduced. This is one of the reasons for the reduction in fluid level. To prove the point further, you will find that, after dieting for a while, whenever you have a drink you will find yourself wanting to pass water very soon afterwards.

It also follows that, if you have a binge (which usually comprises starchy foods), the following day your weight may have risen by as much as 4 pounds (1.75 kilos)! Undoubtedly some of the food which you ate during your gorging session will turn to fat, but not by the next morning! What has happened is that the food you consumed the night before is holding any fluid you may also have consumed, acting rather like a sponge. This is why if, after a binge, you cut down your calories to (say) 1,000 for the next day only, you will find that by the following morning the 4 pounds (1.75 kilos) gained will probably have reduced by 3 pounds (1.5 kilos), leaving the total net damage at only 1 pound (0.5 kilo). And the food you eat weighs a few pounds too. Much of it will eventually be eliminated naturally.

Q. *'If I ate a pound (0.5 kilo) of sausages for my dinner, would I gain a pound (0.5 kilo) in weight if I weighed myself immediately after I had eaten them?'*
A. The answer is yes, providing that you had only just eaten them. There would be no difference in weight whether you ate them or held them in your hand – but only for a few minutes. Because as soon as your body receives food, it begins processing it and using it as fuel.

It's rather like a piece of coal which weighs the same for a few minutes after placing it on the fire as it did before you put it on. But after a while it will begin to burn and disappear except for the waste which remains in the fireplace as ash. If coal were continually being brought in to stoke the fire before it needed it, the coal would have to be stored in something and a coal store would have to be built. Similarly, *we* burn food and excrete any waste – but if we overfeed our bodies we store the excess in fat cells.

Q. *'I get very disheartened when I'm sticking to my diet, yet my weight remains constant or even rises on some days. Why is this?'*
A. It is a mistake to keep popping on to the scales every day – which I suspect you have been doing! The bulk of your body weight is fluid and the level can fluctuate quite alarmingly for no apparent reason, thus giving a very disappointing weight reading. Remember too that most women retain fluid prior to menstruation, or perhaps you haven't had a bowel movement for a day or two – there are hosts of possible explanations.

Another reason for not continually weighing yourself at home is that bathroom scales are, generally speaking, not to be relied upon. If you get on and off them a few times you will find that they give a different reading each time! I wish accurate bathroom scales were available at a reasonable cost, but on the whole they're not. The scales used at my classes are called 'professional' scales and cost around £60. They are the best portable scale I can find – but to get an absolutely accurate weight you need the type of scales which have an arm and a balancing mechanism. We have these at our Head Office and they weigh accurately to within an ounce (25 grams).

I would suggest that you avoid weighing yourself on bathroom scales but make a weekly trip to your chemist, wearing the same clothes each time and weighing yourself at the same time of the day.

Q. *'I'm quite slim except for my thighs. Is there anything I can do to help reduce them? If I diet I lose it from everywhere else – and my bust couldn't get much smaller!'*
A. The number of times I am asked this question! If you really are slim everywhere else, the only solution if your thighs are flabby is a passive exercise machine. Keep-fit exercises or Yoga would certainly help, but I feel that a course of Slendertone or similar treatment would bring faster, more obvious results. Follow the course of treatments with a 'booster' treatment every two or three weeks to keep the problem spot in check.

If you have very firm thighs, then I fear there is little hope. Learn to live with it and stop worrying. Other people won't think the problem is half as serious as you do.

The Helancyl massage glove (available from large stores and chemists) helps to reduce the dimpled effect on legs. You just massage your legs with the glove after your daily bath and then apply their very pleasant-smelling cream. After a month you will begin to see results.

Q. *'I feel so desperate about my weight and I drastically overeat so often I wondered about visiting a hypnotist. What do you think?'*
A. Hypnotists can be very effective in helping some people with certain problems – smoking, over-eating, asthma, etc. But while there is a very high success rate, it is by no means 100 per cent effective.

Consult your own doctor first and discuss the problem with him or her. Your doctor may be able to recommend a reputable hypnotist to you, but you should realise that it may not be the answer to your problem (and hypnosis is expensive).

Acupuncture can also help. A few hypnotists practice acupuncture as well, using the treatments side by side. I have witnessed remarkable successes from this method.

Q. *'I have asked my doctor for some "slimming" pills but she refuses to let me have any as she says they are not the answer to slimming.'*
A. I wholeheartedly agree with your doctor! I'm delighted she has not given you any appetite-suppressant tablets. People who do take them certainly lose their appetite and also lose weight – but they cannot take these tablets for ever, and as soon as they stop they revert to their old eating habits and almost certainly regain all their lost weight.

To lose weight you must learn which foods are good for you and which foods are not; which foods contain fewer calories and which foods are high in calories. You must educate your stomach towards sensible eating during your slimming campaign and afterwards to ensure that you never regain your lost weight.

Q. *'I sometimes eat a "slimmers product" meal in place of ordinary food – is that all right?'*
A. Yes, but I would not encourage anyone to substitute more than one meal a day for this type of food. These products are carefully prepared and are very acceptable if you're crazy about biscuits, milk shakes or chocolate. But remember that, generally speaking, they are not lower in calories than the 'ordinary' comparative food. The difference is that they are fortified with extra vitamins so that you will not suffer any deficiency as a result of eating them in place of an ordinary meal. But this type of food is not helping to re-educate your palate towards healthy food – so I would advise that they should only be included in your diet programme in moderation.
Note The range of products for the slimmer is now very wide.

Frozen 'slimmers' dinners' can be very useful for the house-wife eating on her own during the day and, of course, the food is 'normal'.

Q. *'I should love to visit a health farm. Should I go at the beginning of my slimming campaign or towards the end?'*
A. I would definitely go towards the end – when the going is becoming tough! The treatments will help to tone your body and your stay will make you feel on top of the world as well as helping you lose several pounds (or kilos). But health farms can't work miracles – so if you only go for a week, don't expect to lose a great deal because you won't! Wouldn't it be a wonderful incentive to anyone to slim if someone promised her a week at a health farm when she was within 7 pounds (3 kilos) of her goal weight!

9

You Are *Going To Be Slim*

Think positively! You *are* going to be slim – and by this time next week you will be slimmer than you are today. Here are some of the many benefits *I* experience from being slim:

I feel fitter
 have more confidence in myself
 look much better
 have no problems finding clothes which fit properly
 don't spend as much housekeeping money (with the money I save, I buy extra clothes!)

I love being busy – and now that I have more energy I get loads of work done; before I would spend whole days lounging around doing nothing because I was tired because of overeating because I was bored. A totally vicious circle!

I think the main benefit is that I feel very happy now that I am slim. I used to long to go to bed to get the day over with so that I could start dieting properly tomorrow. Now I wish that there were 48 hours in every day because there is so much that I want to do.

My mind used to be filled with an obsession about being slim and I would hate girls who were slimmer than I. I was for ever comparing myself with the lady over the road who was plump – indeed, with anyone I saw in the town or on television!

Life has been very good to me and I have been very lucky in many, many ways. I'm glad I did something about my weight while I was young because I would have missed so much if I had remained fat. No one is happier when they are overweight and it is never too late to do something about it, so resolve now that you are going to take action. No, not tomorrow, but *now*, this very minute.

You *can* do it and you *will* do it. Decide which diet plan suits you best and write down a shopping list of the various foods you'll need.

Weigh yourself before you start and thereafter just once a week. Record your weekly losses and note any points which might be of interest, such as meals you particularly enjoyed, days when you felt a bit hungry, frequency of cheats, etc. Ask yourself if you felt a greater inclination to cheat if you ate on your own or when you dined with others. This information will add up to an ultimate foolproof programme of eating, just for you.

Write down everything you eat – don't waste time by guessing at how many calories you are eating.

Not only are you going to diet sensibly now – but also resolve that you are going to make the most of your appearance from now on. Aim to keep your hair freshly washed and think before dressing – select something from your wardrobe which you really enjoy wearing. Wear it frequently now as it won't fit you for much longer! Manicure your nails and pay attention to personal hygiene. Take time and trouble with yourself – you're going to be a super new you! Start living again!

In a few weeks you'll find your friends saying: 'Hey, you look terrific – what have you done to yourself? Whatever it is, it really suits you!' Need I say more . . .? Except . . . Good luck!

To find out more about the SSAGG Successful Slimming and Good Grooming Clubs, contact the Head Office:

> The SSAGG Centre,
> Belvoir House,
> 79 Vaughan Way,
> Leicester LE1 4SG.
> *Tel:* Leicester (0533) 538811

10

Recipes

Winter Salad

Serves 1   *60 calories per portion*

1 small tomato
1 small onion, preferably
   Spanish
1 carrot
75g/3oz raw white
   cabbage
¼ green or red pepper
few sprigs raw cauliflower

1 raw mushroom, chopped
pinch of parsley,
   marjoram and chervil
salt and freshly ground
   pepper
juice of ¼ lemon
1 tablespoon cider vinegar

Slice the tomato and finely shred the onion, carrot, cabbage and green or red pepper. Break the cauliflower sprigs into tiny florets. Combine all the vegetables, including the chopped mushroom, and add the herbs and seasonings. Toss in a large bowl with the lemon juice and cider vinegar. Cover and leave in the refrigerator to marinate, preferably for 1½ hours or more.

Savoury Minced Beef

Serves 2   *200 calories per portion*

100g/4oz lean minced
   beef
½ teaspoon mixed herbs
salt and freshly ground
   pepper

1 tablespoon finely
   chopped onion
beaten egg to bind
150ml/¼ pint tomato
   juice

Mix the beef, herbs, salt, pepper and onion together. Bind with the beaten egg. Form into balls. Place in an ovenproof dish and pour over the tomato juice. Bake in a moderate oven (180°C, 350°F, Gas Mark 4) for 45 minutes. Serve with vegetables.

Barbecued Chicken Joints

Serves 2   *200 calories per portion*

2 chicken joints, skinned
1 teaspoon oil
2 tablespoons French
  mustard

2 tablespoons
  Worcestershire sauce
2 tablespoons tomato
  ketchup

Lightly brush the chicken with the oil. Place under the grill
and cook, turning frequently, until almost tender. Mix the
mustard with the Worcestershire sauce and tomato ketchup.
Brush over the chicken joints and continue to grill, basting
occasionally, until crisp and brown. Serve with vegetables or
green salad.

Fruit Meringue

Serves 1   *calorie value depends on fruit used*

75g/3oz fresh fruit purée,
  eg. rhubarb, goose-
  berry or apple (see
  method)

1 egg white, stiffly beaten
liquid artificial sweetener
  to taste

Place the fruit and 2 teaspoons water in a pan and cook until
tender. Rub through a sieve or liquidise. Fold half the stiffly
beaten egg white into the purée and add the artificial
sweetener to taste. Spoon into an ovenproof dish. Place the
remaining egg white on top. Bake in a cool oven (150°C,
300°F, Gas Mark 2) until the meringue is golden.

Slimline Jelly

Serves 4   *12 calories per portion*

15g/½ oz gelatine
  (1 envelope)
600ml/1 pint cold water
50g/2oz blackberries
  (fresh or frozen) or
  similar fruit

10 artificial sweetener
  tablets
squeeze of lemon juice

Soak the gelatine in a little of the water in a pan, off the heat.
Place the fruit and artificial sweetener in another pan with

150ml/¼ pint of the water and simmer gently until the fruit is cooked and the liquid is a good colour. Add the lemon juice and remaining water.

Meanwhile, gently heat the gelatine until dissolved. Pour the cooked fruit on to the gelatine liquid and stir well. Place in 4 individual moulds or dishes, making sure that the fruit is distributed evenly.

Serve with 2 tablespoons top of the milk (16 calories) or 1 tablespoon whipping cream (25 calories).

Lemon Meringue Pie

Serves 4   *112 calories per portion*

2 tablespoons dried
  skimmed milk
300ml/½ pint water
12 artificial sweetener
  tablets

15g/½ oz cornflour
2 eggs, separated
grated rind and juice of
  1 lemon
25g/1oz castor sugar

Mix the dried milk and water together, pour all but 3 tablespoons into a pan and heat until boiling. Add the artificial sweetener. Mix the cornflour to a paste with the reserved cold milk. When the milk is hot, pour on to the cornflour mixture. Return to the pan and bring to the boil, stirring constantly. Leave to cool a little, then stir in the egg yolks and mix well. Add the lemon rind and juice and mix well. Pass the mixture through a sieve, if liked. Pour the mixture into an ovenproof dish. Cook in a moderate oven (160°C, 325°F, Gas Mark 3) for 15 minutes or until set.

Meanwhile, whisk the egg whites until stiff, then fold in the castor sugar. Spoon or pipe the meringue on top of the lemon mixture, return it to the oven and cook until the meringue is golden brown and crisp.

Slimmer's Gâteau

Makes one 20cm/8 inch cake   *130 calories per slice*

3 eggs
130g/4½ oz castor sugar
85g/3oz plain flour

pinch of salt
450g/1 lb eating apples,
  peeled, cored and sliced

88

grated rind and juice of
   1 lemon
1 tablespoon low-calorie
   apricot jam

artificial sweetener
   (optional)
1 teaspoon icing sugar

Grease a 20cm/8 inch cake tin with a butter paper, dust with castor sugar and then dust with flour. Shake out the excess.

Place the eggs and castor sugar in a mixing bowl and whisk with an electric mixer for 5 minutes at top speed. When thick and mousse-like, fold in the sifted flour and salt. Pour into the prepared tin. Bake in the centre of a moderately hot oven (190°C, 375°F, Gas Mark 5) for 25 minutes or until golden brown and shrunk from the edges of the tin a little. Run a blunt knife around the inside of the tin and turn the cake out on to a wire rack to cool.

For the filling, place the apple slices in a pan with the grated lemon rind and juice, and jam. Heat slowly. Add artificial sweetener to taste, if used. Cover and cook until the apples are just tender. When the cake is cool, slice it across with a large knife to make two cakes. Spread the bottom half with the cooled apple filling and cover with the top half of cake. Sprinkle with icing sugar on top.

If you wish, you may cover the top with melted chocolate or with whipped cream, but this obviously adds more calories, which must be taken into account.

Note The total number of calories in an ordinary Victoria Sandwich (3-egg recipe) is approximately 4,224. At 10 slices per cake, each portion contains 422 calories, nearly 300 calories more than a 1/10th portion of Slimmer's Gâteau.

Calorie List

All calorie values are approximate, and this table is only meant to be used as a guide.

Food	Calories	Food	Calories
All Bran, per 25g/1oz	70	Apple Pie, 100g/4oz	220
Alpen, per 2g/1oz	105	Apricots, dried, raw,	
Apple, average (100g/4oz)	40	per 25g/1oz	45
Apple Juice, 100ml/4 fl oz	40	Apricots, fresh, per 25g/1oz	5

Food	Calories	Food	Calories
Apricots, tinned in sugar		Bread, per 25g/1oz	70
syrup, per 25g/1oz	30	Bread, fried	165
Asparagus, 100g/4oz	20	Bread, Nimble or Slimcea	80
Aubergine, per 25g/1oz	4	Broccoli, 100g/4oz	20
Avocado, ½ pear		Brussels Sprouts, 100g/4oz	40
(average)	300	Butter, per 25g/1oz	210
		Butter, Peanut,	
Bacon, fat, grilled,		per 25g/1oz	180
per 25g/1oz	140		
Bacon, lean, grilled,			
per 25g/1oz	100	Cabbage, 100g/4oz	20
Banana, average size,		Carrots, 100g/4oz	20
peeled	80	Cashew Nuts,	
Barley Water, per 25ml/		per 25g/1oz	160
1 fl oz	30	Cauliflower, 100g/4oz	20
Beans, Baked, per 25g/1oz	20	Celery, 100g/4oz	20
Beans, Broad, per 25g/1oz	20	Cheese, Cheddar,	
Beans, Butter, per 25g/1oz	25	per 25g/1oz	120
Beans, French, green or		Cheese, Cottage,	
runner, 100g/4oz	12	per 25g/1oz	30
Bean Sprouts, per 25g/1oz	10	Cheese, Cream,	
Beef, lean, per 25g/1oz	60	per 25g/1oz	150
Beer, 300ml/½ pint	100	Cheese, Double Gloucester	
Beetroot, per 25g/1oz	15	per 25g/1oz	105
Biscuits, Chocolate, each		Cheese, Edam,	
(average)	130	per 25g/1oz	85
Biscuits, plain, each		Cheese, Stilton,	
(average)	50	per 25g/1oz	95
Blackberries, fresh,		Cheesecake, per 25g/1oz	150
per 25g/1oz	10	Cherries, fresh, 100g/4oz	40
Black Pudding, raw,		Cherries, glacé,	
per 25g/1oz	100	per 25g/1oz	60
Blancmange, 100g/4oz		Chestnuts, shelled,	
helping	120	per 25g/1oz	50
Bounty Bar, each bar	140	Chewing Gum, 1 stick	10
Bournvita, per 25g/1oz		Chicken, meat only	
powder	105	per 25g/1oz	50
Bovril, per 25g/1oz (before		Chips, thick-cut,	
adding water)	30	per 25g/1oz	40
Bran, per 25g/1oz	50	Chips, thin crinkle-cut,	
Brandy, per 25ml/1 fl oz	75	per 25g/1oz	75
Brazil Nuts, per 25g/1oz		Chocolate, per 25g/1oz	
(shelled)	178	(approx)	160

Food	Calories	Food	Calories
Chocolate, Drinking, powder, per 25g/1oz	115	Custard powder, per 25g/1oz	100
Christmas Pudding, per 25g/1oz	100	Damsons, fresh, per 25g/1oz	10
Cider, 300ml/½ pint	100	Dates, flesh only, per 25g/1oz	70
Coca Cola, per 25ml/1 fl oz	10	Doughnuts, per 25g/1oz (average)	100
Cocoa Powder, per 25g/1oz	95	Dripping, beef, per 25g/1oz	250
Coconut, dessicated, per 25g/1oz	170	Duck, roast, per 25g/1oz	90
Coconut, fresh, per 25g/1oz	100	Eels, jellied, per 25g/1oz	105
Cod, Cutlet, fried, per 25g/1oz	50	Egg, one, boiled or poached	90
Cod, Cutlet, steamed, per 25g/1oz	25	Egg, one, fried	135
Coffee	nil	Egg, one, omelette or scrambled	100
Coffeemate, per 25g/1oz	160	Egg, Scotch, average size	250
Coleslaw, 50g/2oz	80	Energen Rolls, per roll	25
Complan, per 25g/1oz	120	Faggots, per 25g/1oz (average)	80
Corn on the Cob, fresh, boiled, per 25g/1oz	34	Figs, dried, per 25g/1oz	60
Corned Beef, per 25g/1oz	65	Figs, fresh, per 25g/1oz	10
Cornflakes, per 25g/1oz	105	Figs, tinned, per 25g/1oz	55
Cornflour, powder, per 25g/1oz	100	Fish, white, steamed, per 25g/1oz (average)	30
Country Store, per 25g/1oz	105	Fish Cakes, per 25g/1oz	35
Courgettes, 100g/4oz	20	Fish Fingers, each	55
Crab, 50g/2oz meat only	70	Flora Margarine, per 25g/1oz	210
Cream, fresh, double per 25ml/1 fl oz	130	Flour, per 25g/1oz	100
Cream, single, per 25ml/1 fl oz	60	Frankfurter Sausages, per 25g/1oz	70
Cream, top of the milk per 25ml/1 fl oz	55	Fruit Cake, per 25g/1oz (average)	120
Cream, whipping per 25ml/1 fl oz	100	Fruit Salad, fresh, per 25g/1oz (average)	20
Cress, fresh, per 25g/1oz	4	Fudge, 100g/4oz	480
Crisps, 25g/1oz packet	145		
Crispbreads, 1 (average)	25	Gammon Ham, per 25g/1oz	60
Cucumber, per 25g/1oz	5		

Food	Calories	Food	Calories
Gherkins	neg	Ice Cream, per 25g/1oz	60
Ginger Ale, American, per 25ml/1 fl oz	10	Ideal Milk, per 25ml/1 fl oz	45
Ginger Ale, Slimline	neg	Instant Whip, as served, per 25g/1oz	30
Ginger Biscuits, per 25g/1oz	125	Jam, per 25g/1oz (average)	80
Glucose, per 25g/1oz	110		
Gold, per 25g/1oz	105	Jam, Energen low-calorie, per 25g/1oz	50
Gooseberries, fresh, raw, per 25g/1oz	10	Jam Tarts, short pastry, per 25g/1oz	110
Grapes, black, fresh per 25g/1oz	18	Jelly (not made up), per 25g/1oz	80
Grapes, green, fresh per 25g/1oz	18		
Grapefruit, fresh, per 25g/1oz	5	Ketchup, Tomato, per 25g/1oz	30
Grapefruit, tinned in sugar syrup, per 25g/1oz	18	Kidneys, per 25g/1oz	40
		Kipper, fillet, per 25g/1oz	60
Grapefruit, juice, unsweetened, per 25ml/1 fl oz	10	Lager, 300ml/½ pint (approx.)	100
Grapenuts, per 25g/1oz	100	Lamb Chop, grilled, per 25g/1oz	60
Guinness, 300ml/½ pint	100		
		Lamb Chop, roast, fat, per 25g/1oz	80
Haddock, fresh, steamed, per 25g/1oz	30	Lamb Chop, roast, lean, per 25g/1oz	55
Haddock, fried, per 25g/1oz	50	Lard, per 25g/1oz	255
Haggis, per 25g/1oz	50	Leek, 100g/4oz	30
Ham, fat and lean, per 25g/1oz	110	Lemon, fresh, per 25g/1oz	5
		Lemon Curd, per 25g/1oz	85
Ham, lean, per 25g/1oz	60	Lemon Drink, low-calorie	neg
Hamburger, per 25g/1oz	80	Lemon juice, unsweetened, per 25ml/1 fl oz	5
Hazlet, per 25g/1oz	80		
Heart, Sheep's, roast, per 25g/1oz	70	Lemonade, 300ml/½ pint	50
Herring, per 25g/1oz	50	Lentils, boiled, per 25g/1oz	25
Honey, per 25g/1oz (average)	100	Lettuce, per 25g/1oz	5
		Lime Cordial, per 25g/1oz	30
Horlicks, powder per 25g/1oz	120	Liquorice, per 25g/1oz	100
Horseradish Sauce, per 25g/1oz	25	Liver, per 25g/2oz (average)	50
		Liver Pâté, per 25g/1oz	140

Food	Calories	Food	Calories
Liver Sausage, per 25g/1oz	85	Melon, yellow, fresh (no skin) per 25g/1oz	4
Lobster, fresh, boiled per 25g/1oz	35	Milk, condensed sweetened, per 25ml/1 fl oz	95
Loganberries, fresh, per 25g/1oz	5	Milk, evaporated, per 25ml/1 fl oz	45
Loganberries, tinned in sugar syrup, per 25g/1oz (average)	30	Milk, fresh, silver top, 300ml/½ pint	185
Lucozade, per 25ml/1 fl oz	22	Milk, reconstituted skimmed, 300ml/½ pint	100
Luncheon Meat, per 25g/1oz	80	Mincemeat, per 25g/1oz	38
Macaroni, boiled per 25g/1oz	30	Mint Sauce (with sugar), 25g/1oz	40
Macaroni Cheese, per 25g/1oz	55	Muesli, per 25g/1oz	105
Mackerel, fillet, fried, per 25g/1oz	55	Mushrooms, boiled, grilled or raw, per 25g/1oz	5
Mandarin Oranges, fresh per 25g/1oz	10	Mushrooms, fried, per 15g/1oz	50
Mandarin Oranges, tinned in sugar syrup, per 25g/1oz	20	Mustard, made, per 25g/1oz	120
Margarine, per 25g/1oz (average)	210	Mustard Cress, raw, per 25g/1oz	4
Marmalade, per 25g/1oz (average)	75	Nimble bread, per slice	40
Marmalade, Energen low-calorie, per 25g/1oz	50	Oats (Porridge), dry, per 25g/1oz	115
Marmite, per 25g/1oz	33	Oil, cooking, vegetable, per 25ml/1 fl oz	250
Marrow, boiled or baked without fat, per 25g/1oz	neg	Olive Oil, per 25ml/1 fl oz	260
Mars Bar, whole bar	300	Omelette, 2 eggs, no fat	200
Martini, dry, per 25ml/1 fl oz	35	Onion, boiled or raw, per 25g/1oz	5
Martini Bianco, per 25ml/1 fl oz	45	Onion, fried, per 25g/1oz	100
Marvel, made up, 300ml/½ pint	100	Orange, fresh (average)	50
Mayonnaise (real), per 25g/1oz	160	Orange Juice, per 25ml/1 fl oz	10
		Outline, per 25g/1oz	110
		Ovaltine, powder, per 25g/1oz	110
		Oxo, 1 cube	11
		Oxtail, per 25g/1oz	30

Food	Calories	Food	Calories
Ox Tongue, per 25g/1oz	90	Pizza, per 25g/1oz (average)	65
Oysters, per 25g/1oz	15		
Pancakes, fried, per 25g/1oz	85	Plaice, fried in breadcrumbs, per 25g/1oz	60
Parsnip, boiled, per 25g/1oz	15	Plaice, steamed, per 25g/1oz	20
Parsnip, roast, per 25g/1oz	35	PLJ (pure lemon juice), per 25ml/1 fl oz	5
Passion Fruit, fresh, per 25g/1oz	5	Plums, fresh, per 25g/1oz	10
Pasta, per 25g/1oz	95	Plums, tinned in sugar syrup, per 25g/1oz	20
Pastry, cooked, per 25g/1oz (average)	140	Pomagne, dry, per 25ml/1 fl oz	16
Pâté, per 25g/1oz (average)	135	Pomagne, sweet, per 25ml/1 fl oz	20
Peach, fresh, raw, per 25g/1oz	10	Polo Mints, 1 pack	90
Peaches, tinned in sugar syrup, per 25g/1oz	22	Pork, grilled, lean, per 25g/1oz	90
Peanuts, salted, per 25g/1oz	165	Pork, roast, lean and fat per 25g/1oz	130
Peanut Butter, per 25g/1oz	175	Pork Pie, per 25g/1oz	110
Pear, fresh, 100g/4oz (average)	40	Porridge (Oats), dry, per 25g/1oz	115
Pears, tinned, in sugar syrup, per 25g/1oz	20	Port Wine, 60ml/2¼ fl oz (average glass)	100
Peas, per 25g/1oz	20	Potato, jacket, per 25g/1oz	25
Peppers, green or red, per 25g/1oz	5	Potato, new, boiled, per 25g/1oz	20
Pheasant, roast, meat only, per 25g/1oz	65	Potato, old, boiled per 25g/1oz	25
Pickle, Branston per 25g/1oz	35	Potato, roast, per 25g/1oz	35
Pickled Onions, Gherkins, etc., per 25g/1oz	2	Potato Chips, large, per 25g/1oz	40
Pilchards, tinned, per 25g/1oz	50	Potato Chips, narrow, crinkle-cut, per 25g/1oz	75
Pineapple, fresh, raw, per 25g/1oz	12	Potato Crisps, 25g/1oz packet	150
Pineapple, tinned in sugar syrup, per 25g/1oz	20	Prawns, per 25g/1oz (shelled)	30

Food	Calories	Food	Calories
Prunes, stewed (no sugar), per 25g/1oz	20	Sauces, thick, per 25ml/1 fl oz (average)	100
Puffed Wheat, per 25g/1oz	105	Sauces, thin, per 25ml/1 fl oz (average)	25
Pumpkin, fresh, per 25g/1oz	5	Sausage, beef, 50g/2oz (average)	190
		Sausage, frankfurter, 50g/2oz	140
Rabbit, roast or stewed, per 25g/1oz	50	Sausage, pork, 50g/2oz (average)	190
Raisins, dried, 25g/1oz	80	Sausage Rolls, per 25g/1oz	100
Raisin Bran, per 25g/1oz	100	Scanda Crisp, 1 biscuit	22
Raspberries, fresh, per 25g/1oz	5	Scone, per 25g/1oz (average)	95
Raspberries, tinned in sugar syrup, per 25g/1oz	25	Scotch Egg, average size	250
Ravioli, per 25g/1oz	30	Semolina, before cooking, per 25g/1oz	100
Rhubarb, stewed (no sugar), per 25g/1oz	2	Shellfish, per 25g/1oz (average)	25
Ribena, per 25ml/1 fl oz	85	Sherry, dry, per 25ml/1 fl oz	30
Rice, before cooking, per 25g/1oz	100	Sherry, sweet, per 25ml/1 fl oz	35
Rice Krispies, per 25g/1oz	100	Shredded Wheat, per 25g/1oz	115
Roe, cod or herring, fried, (approx.)	70	Shreddies, per 25g/1oz	115
Rolls, usually 50g/2oz	140	Shrimps, per 25g/1oz	30
Ryvita, 1 biscuit	27	Skate, fried, per 25g/1oz	60
		Slimcea bread, per slice	40
Sago, before cooking, per 25g/1oz	100	Sole, steamed, per 25g/1oz	25
Salad Cream, per 25g/1oz	110	Soups (depending on thickness)	5-30
Salad Cream, low-calorie, per 25g/1oz	50	Soya Flour, per 25g/1oz	125
Salami, per 25g/1oz	115	Soya Protein, per 25g/1oz (average)	65
Salmon, fresh, per 25g/1oz	55	Spinach, 100g/4oz	20
Salmon, tinned, per 25g/1oz	45	Spirits (alcoholic), per 25ml/1 fl oz	70
Sandwich Spread, per 25g/1oz (average)	50	Squash, Fruit, concentrated, per 25ml/1 fl oz	40
Sardines, tinned, per 25g/1oz	60		

Food	Calories	Food	Calories
Steak, grilled, per 25g/1oz	50	Trout, steamed on bone, per 25g/1oz	30
Strawberries, fresh, per 25g/1oz	5	Tuna, tinned, per 25g/1oz	65
Strawberries, tinned in sugar syrup, per 25g/1oz	20	Turbot, steamed, per 25g/1oz	30
Suet, per 25g/1oz	240	Turkey, roast, meat only, per 25g/1oz	45
Sugar, 1 teaspoon (average)	20	Turnip, boiled, per 25g/1oz	5
Sugar, per 25g/1oz	110		
Sugar Puffs, per 25g/1oz	105	Veal, in breadcrumbs, per 25g/1oz	65
Sultanas, per 25g/1oz	75		
Swedes, boiled, 100g/4oz	20	Waistline Salad Dressing, per 25ml/1 fl oz	50
Sweetcorn, 100g/4oz	120	Walnuts, per 25g/1oz, (shelled)	150
Sweetex, tablets or liquid	nil		
Syrup (Golden), per 25ml/1 fl oz	90	Watercress, fresh, raw, per 25g/1oz	4
		Weetabix, each	55
Tangarines, fresh, per 25g/1oz	10	Whisky, 25ml/1 fl oz	65
Tangarines, tinned in sugar syrup, per 25g/1oz	18	Whitebait, fried, per 25g/1oz	150
Tea	neg	Wine, average dry, per 25ml/1 fl oz	20
Tomato, fresh, per 25g/1oz	5	Wine, average sweet, per 25ml/1 fl oz	25
Tomato, fried, per 25g/1oz	20		
Tomato Ketchup, per 25g/1oz	30	Yeast, fresh, per 25g/1oz	20
Tongue, Ox or Sheep, per 25g/1oz	85	Yoghurt, fruit-flavoured 150g/5oz carton	125
Tonic Water, Schweppes, 200ml/7 fl oz	70	Yoghurt, natural 150g/5oz carton	60
Tonic Water, Schweppes, Slimline	neg	Yorkshire Pudding, per 25g/1oz	60
Tripe, per 25g/1oz	30		